# VETERINARY MANAGEMENT OF TORTOISES AND TURTLES



**Stuart McArthur**
MRCVS

Blackwell
Science

Editorial Offices:
Osney Mead, Oxford OX2 0EL
25 John Street, London WC1N 2BL
23 Ainslie Place, Edinburgh EH3 6AJ
238 Main Street, Cambridge,
Massachusetts 02142, USA
54 University Street, Carlton,
Victoria 3053, Australia

Other Editorial Offices:
Arnette Blackwell SA
1, rue de Lille, 75007 Paris
France

Blackwell Wissenschafts-Verlag GmbH
Kurfürstendamm 57
10707 Berlin, Germany

Feldgasse 13, A-1238 Wien
Austria



First published 1996

Set in 10/13pt Melior
by DP Photosetting, Aylesbury, Bucks
Printed and bound at the
Alden Press, Oxford

DISTRIBUTORS

Marston Book Services Ltd
PO Box 87
Oxford OX2 0DT
(*Orders:* Tel: 01865 791155
Fax: 01865 791927
Telex: 837515)

USA
Blackwell Science, Inc.
238 Main Street
Cambridge, MA 02142
(*Orders:* Tel: 800 215-1000
617 876-7000
Fax: 617 492-5263)

Canada
Oxford University Press
70 Wynford Drive
Don Mills
Ontario M3C 1J9
(*Orders:* Tel: 416 441 2941)

Australia
Blackwell Science Pty Ltd
54 University Street
Carlton, Victoria 3053
(*Orders:* Tel: 03 347-0300
Fax: 03 349-3016)

A catalogue record for this title
is available from the British Library

ISBN 0–632–04059–9

Library of Congress
Cataloging-in-Publication Data
McArthur, Stuart.
Veterinary management of tortoises and turtles/Stuart McArthur.
Includes bibliographical references and index.
ISBN 0–632–04059–9 (alk. paper)
1. Turtles—Diseases. I. Title.
SF997.5.T87M38 1995
639.3′92—dc20 95-38446
CIP

# CONTENTS

# PREFACE

This book aims to provide general practice veterinarians with an accurate and easy to use manual of tortoise and turtle conditions. Tables and note format have been used wherever possible in order to assist with quick reference.

The book deals with many medical and surgical conditions and tries to include photographs and illustrations to help to keep this information clear. Advice concerning hibernation, laboratory tests, anatomy, the management of egg retention and information such as the drugs and doses used in treating Chelonia have also been included. It is hoped that a veterinarian will be able to tackle most situations with the information provided.

There are currently about 240 different species of Chelonia and they vary greatly in size, diet and environmental tolerances. This book concentrates on those species commonly encountered in captivity in the UK and does not specifically deal with wild species, although most of the information included will be relevant to those as well.

Whilst many of the treatment options given are only suggestions, they should provide a safe and useful starting point for most situations. The most appropriate management of specific conditions has to be somewhat subjective. The literature available often deals with small numbers of animals and it is known that opinions within veterinary circles can vary to the extreme. It is difficult to conduct controlled treatment trials with endangered species kept in varying conditions of husbandry.

This book has reviewed a large amount of the literature available and it has been repeatedly modified on the advice of fellow veterinarians. Husbandry information has been offered by experienced individuals who manage tortoise welfare, breeding and conservation projects.

The book is the result of the co-operation and effort of a large team of individuals interested in the welfare of these interesting but endangered animals. I am very grateful to all concerned. Opinions relate to my own personal experience and are given to complement those of the veterinarian using the manual.

## DISCLAIMER

Whilst every effort has been taken to ensure the products suggested and the drug doses advised in this text are both safe and effective, veterinarians are reminded that no responsibility is taken by the author or publisher from any matter that may arise as a result of their administration to an animal. The information given was up-to-date at the time of writing.

There are no obvious medical products that are specifically licensed for use in Chelonia so I have tried to list as wide a variety of drugs as possible suitable for them. This has drawn on the literature cited in the Bibliography and preparations used previously by the author. Often the brand name is also included but this does not mean that other preparations would not be equally effective. Current indexes and compendiums of veterinary drugs should be consulted.

Veterinarians should take their own precautions to ensure that new legislation, such as the recent Cascade introduced after this book was written, is followed wherever possible. It may be wise to use a form such as that issued by the Veterinary Defence Society to obtain consent from the client before administration.

# ACKNOWLEDGEMENTS

My greatest thanks go to Andy Highfield who has suffered a lot of stress in his efforts to ensure this book was both accurate and of a high standard. He has helped me greatly over the past six years and made the book possible by his dedication to Chelonia welfare issues. He has kindly supplied Plates 4, 7–13 and 15.

I would like to thank the British Small Animal Veterinary Association for permission to reproduce Fig. 11.

All the following have helped read the text and have passed on advice. They are not responsible for any errors included and the opinions expressed are not necessarily theirs: The Tortoise Trust, BM Tortoise, London WC1N 3XX; T. Miller MRCVS and Mrs E. Miller; A. Routh MRCVS (of Sea Turtle Survival); A.W. Sainsbury MRCVS (of London Zoo and The World Association of Wildlife Veterinarians); N. Carmichael MRCVS, Grange Laboratories, PO Box 4, Wetherby, LS22 4ZR; David Williams MRCVS (of the RVC); Andrew Greenwood MRCVS (of the International Zoo Veterinary Group); Pip Boydell MRCVS (of the Animal Medical Centre); and Jeremy Fletcher MRCVS.

I would also like to thank Steve Terry for helping with the graphs, Kate Mcguire for the excellent line drawings and Ian Clenshaw for scanning and labelling Kate's pictures.

# ANATOMY

It is the aim of this section to give a basic knowledge of the anatomy of the tortoise, so that the terminology used later is understood. Should the opportunity to perform a post-mortem examination arise, the material gathered is invaluable.

I have included line drawings of the external anatomy of the tortoise (Figs 1–3) and photographs of a dissection of a Mediterranean tortoise (Plates 1–3). Serial removal of viscera has been performed in order to reveal as much of the internal anatomy as possible. Line drawings of the area occupied by the lung fields are included later (Fig. 19).

| Anatomical term | Interpretation |
|---|---|
| **Carapace** | The upper shell of the tortoise |
| **Plastron** | The lower shell of the tortoise |
| **Scutes** | The horny plates of a tortoises shell |
| Vertebral | Central row of scutes along the carapace spine |
| Costal/Plural | Scutes between the vertebrals and marginal |
| Marginal | The scutes along the carapace edge (usually 11) |
| Nuchal | Central carapace scute above head (marginal) |
| Gular | Plastral scute below head |
| Supracaudal | Carapace scute above tail |
| Inguinal | Small triangular scute cranial to hind leg |
| Humoral | Plastral scute behind gular |
| Pectoral | Plastral scute behind humeral |
| Abdominal | Plastral scute behind pectoral |
| Femoral | Plastral scute between anal and abdominal |
| Anal | Last plastral scute, below tail |
| **Suture** | The 'seam' between horny plates |
| **External nares** | Paired nasal openings |
| **Beak** | Horny tissue covering jaws |
| **Scale** | Horny plates of the skin |
| **Tympanic scale** | The scale overlying the ear |
| **Cloaca** | The chamber where urogenital and digestive systems empty |
| **Hinge (plastron)** | A mobile suture in the plastron (e.g. box turtle) |
| **Hinge (carapace)** | A mobile suture in caudal carapace (e.g. hingeback) |

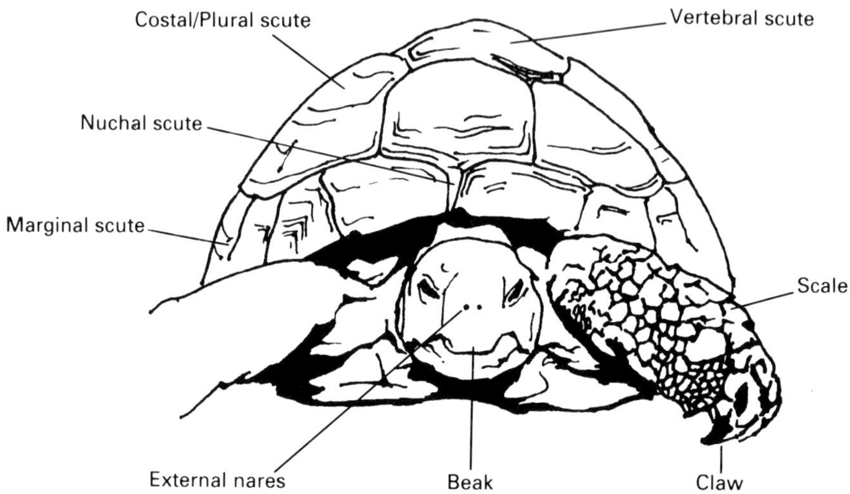


**Fig. 1** The external anatomy of *Testudo hermanni* (anterior view).

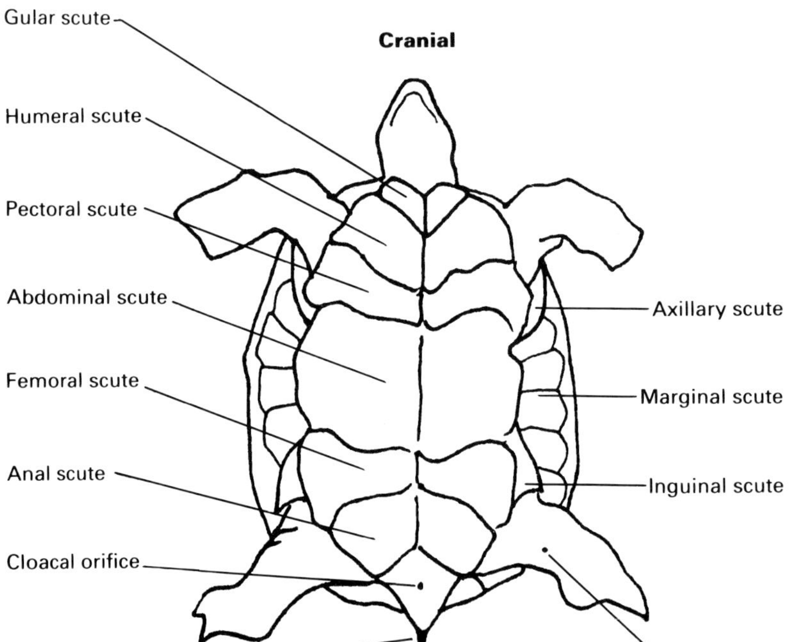


**Fig. 2** A view of the ventral plastron.

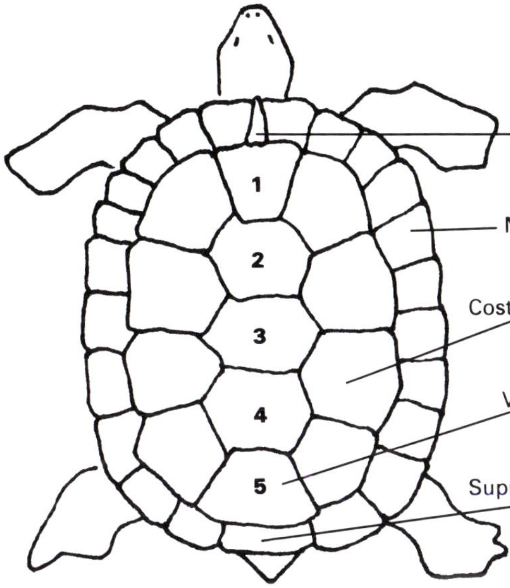


**Fig. 3** A view of the dorsal carapace.

## Serial dissection of a Mediterranean tortoise demonstrating the internal anatomy of a chelonian (Plates 1–3)

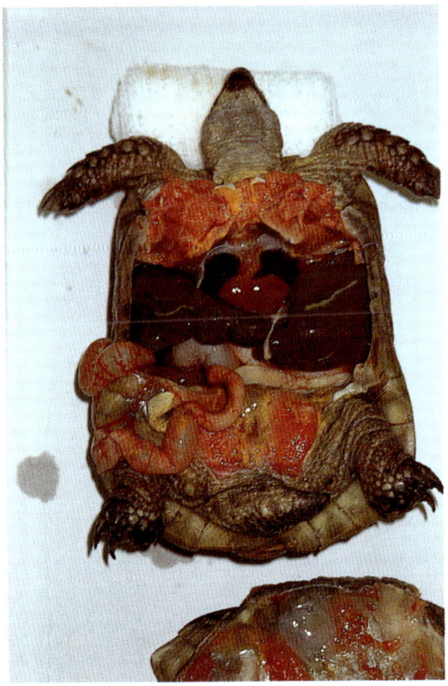

**Plate 1** Dorsal view of the tortoise with plastron removed. This demonstrates the large pelvic and thoracic limb muscle masses, the liver, heart, spleen and small intestine. A kidney is also visible.

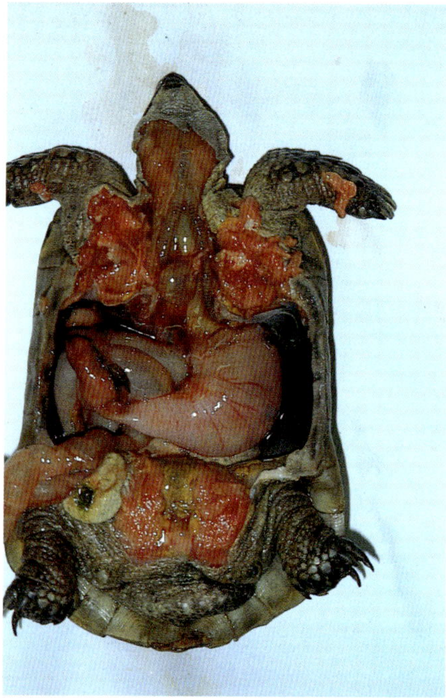

**Plate 2** Further dissection and removal of liver and musclature. This reveals the stomach, large intestine, bifurcated trachea and thyroid gland. The dark lung tissue can be seen lying dorsally.

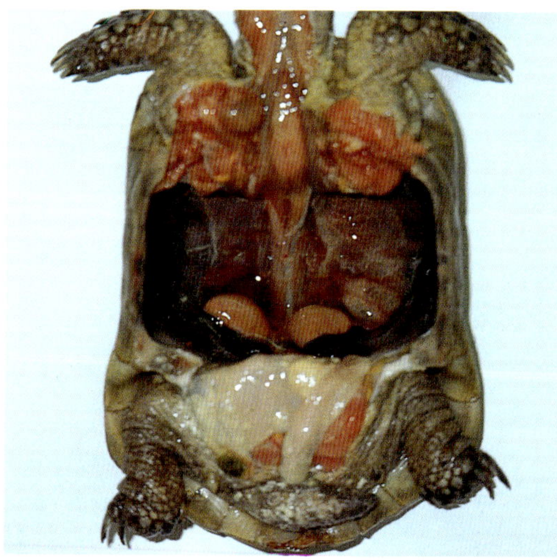

**Plate 3** With the intestines now removed, the two kidneys and bladder (reflected) become obvious lying on top of the darker dorsally positioned lung tissue.

# CLINICAL EXAMINATION

As tortoises are ectotherms and encased in a protective shell it can prove very difficult to give an effective clinical examination. Temperature measurements and auscultation are largely inappropriate, so more importance must be placed on weight, length, and the careful visual examination of all available areas. The general demeanour (activity, eating patterns, etc.) of the tortoise should be assessed in relation to its stage of yearly activity. A full history including nutrition, environment and contact with other tortoises should be taken. Any previous diagnoses and treatment should also be noted. A suggested history/examination form is included later in Appendix 2.

## WEIGH AND MEASURE THE TORTOISE (see Fig. 4)

This is discussed in more detail in the section dealing with hibernation. Specific information has only been published for Mediterranean species, as far as I am aware. Jackson (1980b) demonstrated that when a large number of tortoises of varying length and weight were considered, a graphical representation could be used to show how an individual related to the expected range for the species. A graph of this nature has been included later, see Fig. 11. Caution should be taken in assessing the health of an animal purely on these criteria. It is possible for animals of acceptable weight to be seriously ill. The shortcomings of this information are also demonstrated later under 'the interpretation of weight/length measurements' in the section on 'Hibernation'.

## EXAMINE THE TORTOISE

A sample history/examination form is included in Appendix 2. It may help ensure common conditions are not overlooked.

The following table also summarizes the common presenting symptoms of many tortoise diseases and can act as a simple check list. Plate 4 shows symptoms that may be indicative of several illnesses.

| Region | Possible presenting signs |
|---|---|
| **Eyes** | • Swelling<br>• Discharge<br>• Infections<br>• Cataract<br>• Evidence of vitamin A deficiency<br>• Foreign body, corneal lesions<br>• Jaundice |
| **Ears** | • Swelling and abscess formation<br>• Secondary spread of infection |
| **Mouth** | • Erythema<br>• Haemorrhagic foci<br>• Necrosis<br>• Jaundice<br>• Caseation |
| **Nose** | • Mucus discharge<br>• Purulent discharge<br>• Beak overgrowth |
| **Skin** | • Sloughing<br>• Exudation<br>• Oedema<br>• Abscess formation<br>• Jaundice<br>• Other inflammation<br>• Trauma |
| **Shell** | • Trauma or damage<br>• Infection<br>• Discharge (as in ulcerative shell disease)<br>• The red flush associated with septicaemia |
| **Cloaca** | • Trauma, discharge or infection |

## LABORATORY SAMPLES AND FURTHER INVESTIGATIONS

- **Faeces and urine** may be examined for parasites.
- **Swabs** may be cultured from suspected bacterial infections.
- **Blood** may be taken and biochemistry and haematology assessed.
- **Radiography** if egg retention, calculus formation, pneumonia or limb fracture is suspected.

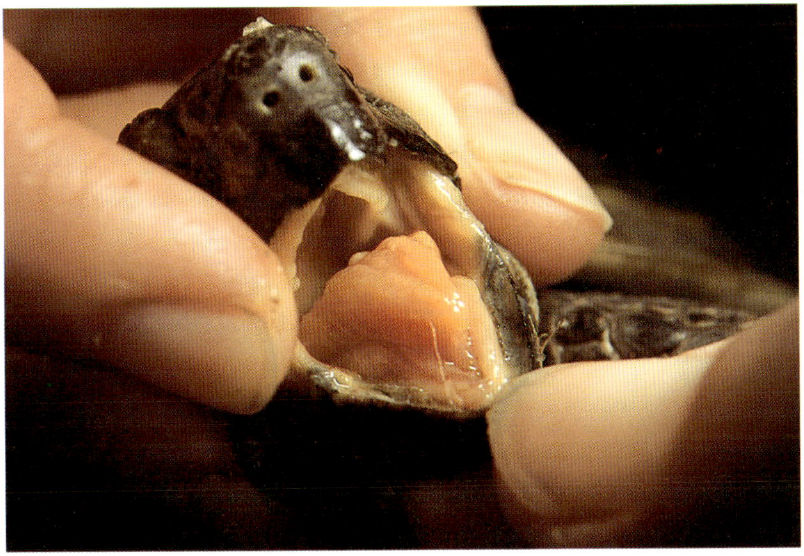

**Plate 4** Jaundiced mouth of *Testudo graeca* with hepatitis. (© A.C. Highfield.)

# HANDLING, INJECTION AND FEEDING TECHNIQUES

## WEIGHING AND MEASURING A MEDITERRANEAN TORTOISE

This is essential during any clinical examination of a Mediterranean tortoise. Weighing is easy if small electronic kitchen scales are used. An active tortoise can be immobilized by placing it on top of a small empty pill container so that its legs cannot reach the ground.

Measurements of carapace length are made easy by using a clear plastic ruler. The distance from front to back of the carapace is measured by eye whilst standing over the animal. The length recorded does not

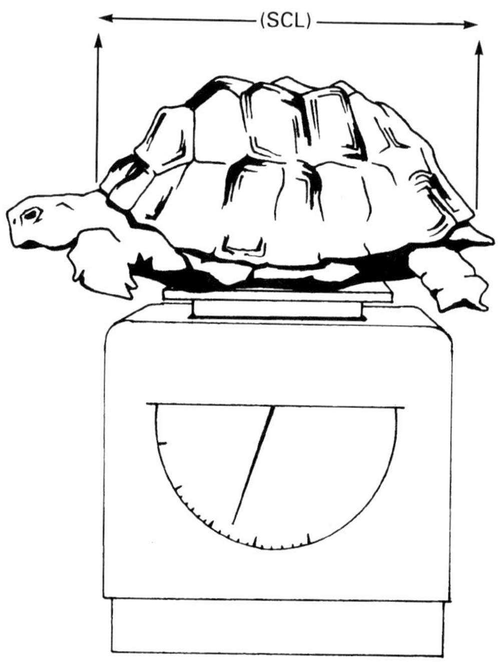


**Fig. 4** Weighing and measuring the tortoise. Straight carapace length (SCL) should be taken in millimetres. Measure in a straight line – do not bend ruler over the curve.

include the upward curvature of the shell and is called the ***straight carapace length*** (SCL). This is usually measured in millimetres (mm), see Fig. 4.

These measurements can be used to compare Mediterranean tortoises to others of the same species using Jackson's graph, a sample of which is included (Fig. 11). This graph is discussed later in the 'Hibernation' section.

## ACCESS TO THE HEAD FOR EXAMINATION

This is accomplished by using a finger either side of the jaw to restrain the head. The other hand can then open the mouth. Shy tortoises will often expose their heads if the clinician is both quick and patient – a gentle tickle of the chin or perineum may help. Sometimes a tortoise will produce its head if a blunt instrument such as a cat urethral catheter is used to gently stimulate its tympanic scale. In extreme cases protected whelping forceps may be of use but care must be taken to prevent injury or distress to the animal.

## SWABBING THE ORAL CAVITY

This is easiest with the animal held upright by an assistant. One hand holds the head extended and mouth open with thumb and forefinger either side of the temporomandibular joint whilst the other hand holds the swab (Fig. 5).

## ACCESS TO A BOX TURTLE FOR EXAMINATION

Box turtles can bite or trap fingers in their box as it is forcibly closed. Their hinged plastron makes a clinical examination much more difficult than with Mediterranean tortoises. The application of pressure to the posterior plastron generally allows the anterior plastron to be opened. If the animal is strong a rubber eraser may be inserted to limit its retreat. The limbs and head can usually be drawn out one after another for examination whilst an assistant squeezes the posterior plastron.

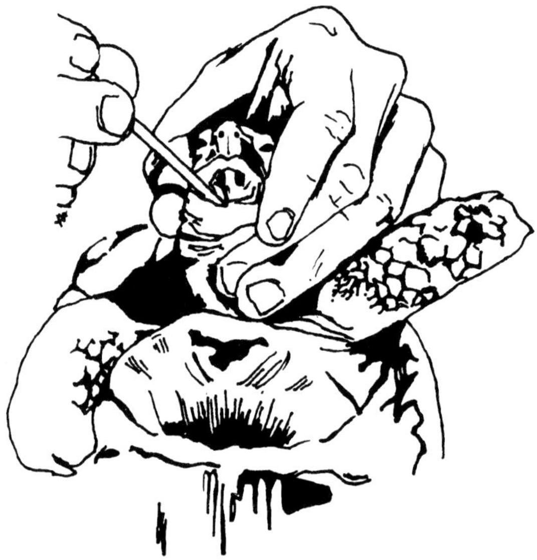

**Fig. 5** Swabbing the oral cavity. A sterile swab can be taken in order to undertake culture and sensitivity testing in cases of necrotic stomatitis. A cotton bud or swab can also be used to debride such an infection and to apply local treatment such as povidone-iodine solution.

## INTRAVENOUS (I.V.) INJECTIONS AND BLOOD SAMPLING

| | |
|---|---|
| **Smaller animals (up to 130 mm)** | • An insulin syringe with a 23 or 25 gauge needle is often suitable. |
| **Average animals (above 130 mm)** | • A 21, 23 or 25 gauge needle on a 2 or 5 ml syringe is usually suitable. |

The site of venepuncture is normally the dorsal tail venous sinus which is found in the midline and runs from virtually the tip of the tail to the junction of the perineum and carapace (Fig. 6).

Insert the needle slowly whilst applying suction. If the sinus is unyielding or not located then one can work more proximally. A tortoise that refuses to expose its tail can often be blood sampled by inserting the needle blind, at the junction of the carapace and perineum in the midline.

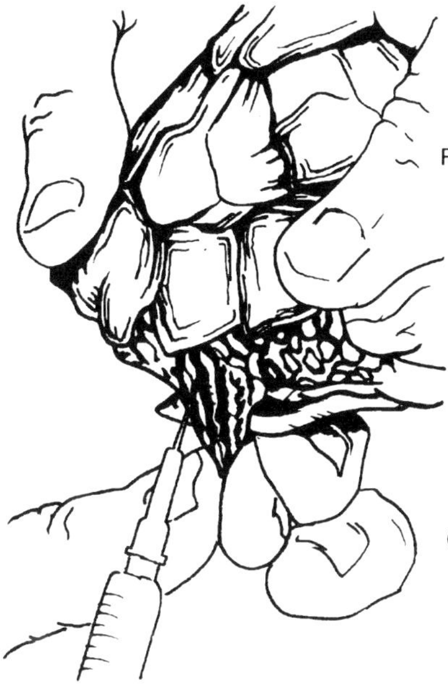


**Fig. 6** Site of intravenous injection or blood sampling. Using the dorsal venous sinus of the tail.

## INTRAMUSCULAR (I.M.) INJECTIONS

Most injections of antibiotics and vitamins will be intramuscular (i.m.) as these preparations tend to be more irritant if given subcutaneously (see Fig. 7).

| | |
|---|---|
| **Hind limb** | • The site is usually the quadriceps mass of the hind leg or the gluteal area. |
| **Fore limb** | • The site is usually the proximal cranial muscle mass of the foreleg. Drugs which may have nephrotoxic qualities may be best given by this route to prevent renal blood levels rising quickly. As a portal system transports blood from the hind limbs through the kidneys. |

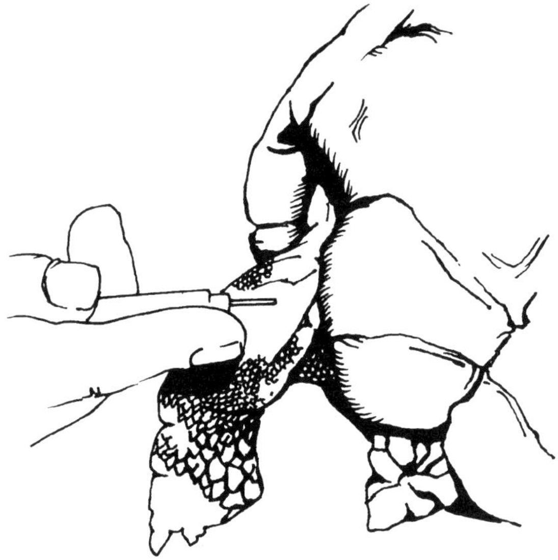

**Fig. 7** Intramuscular injection. The needle is passed into the cranial muscle mass of the hind limb.

## ALTERNATIVE METHODS OF BLOOD SAMPLING, I.V. INJECTIONS AND FLUID THERAPY IN A TORTOISE

| | |
|---|---|
| **Short clipping a nail** | • To provide a small sample of blood for use with an 'Azostix' blood urea test, or similar. |
| **Cardiocentesis** | • This involves drilling a small hole in the plastron. ***As this is an invasive technique it could result in serious complications. I do not advise this myself but it has been employed in some surveys abroad.*** |
| **Jugular venepuncture** | • The tortoise is usually in dorsal recumbency with the head and neck extended.<br>• Small intravenous catheters, 21 gauge or smaller, can be employed.<br>• The volume given or taken in ml on any one occasion should never exceed 5% of the total body weight of the patient in grams (Page & Mautino 1990).<br>• This technique is described by several authors for both blood sampling and intravenous injection of agents such as anaesthetics (Frye 1991; Page & Mautino 1990).<br>• Apparently a better haematology sample can be obtained in this way, in tropical species, as red blood cells tend to haemolyse in samples taken from the dorsal tail venous sinus. |

| | |
|---|---|
| **Intracoelomic injections** | • Intracoelomic fluids can be injected slowly just cranial to the hind limb.<br>• Beware of direct infusion into the bladder and compression of lung tissue by over hydration – do not give greater than 3% of the body weight in ml – (Page & Mautino 1990).<br>• An intracoelomic route, just caudal to the shoulder joint and dorsal to the plastron, has also been described. |

## FORCE FEEDING TORTOISES

Tortoises suffering visual impairment or infections, and tortoises over-wintered at suboptimal temperatures and with poor illumination, may well find feeding by themselves difficult or impossible. Such animals will probably require force feeding if they are to survive. Animals with uncomplicated post-hibernation anorexia (PHA) will also require force feeding.

| | |
|---|---|
| **Hand feeding** | • This requires food to be actively placed in the tortoise's mouth. Small blunt-ended forceps are suitable here and the food offered should be the diet described elsewhere under 'Nutrition'. Tortoises suffering from temperature related visual impairment and similar conditions, may respond well to this husbandry and given some considerable time may regain sight to a degree. |
| **Syringe feeding** | • A small amount of liquid or liquidized food is squirted into the tortoise's mouth. This is best done by giving small amounts frequently. |

## STOMACH TUBING AND ORAL DOSING A TORTOISE

Worming preparations, fluids and liquidized foods are often delivered via a stomach tube. Various instruments and tubes can be used but I tend to use a Jackson Cat Catheter (4 French gauge or larger) or a suitable dog urethral catheter lubricated at the end and marked to about half the length of the plastron, so one can judge how close to the stomach it is (Fig. 8). A 2, 5, 10 or 20 ml syringe can be attached to the Luer tip and the contents slowly administered.

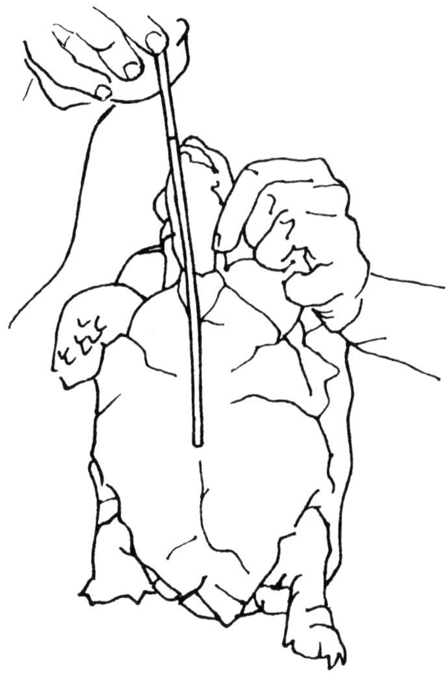

**Fig. 8** Measuring a stomach tube. This is easiest with the tortoise held upright with its neck in extension. A suitable stomach tube, such as a dog urethral catheter, is marked from the chin to the middle of the plastron.

The tube is easiest passed with an assistant holding the tortoise in an upright position, facing the person who is passing the stomach tube. Before passing a stomach tube ensure that it is already filled with an appropriate liquid, otherwise a lot of air will be placed directly into the stomach when the syringe is attached.

In mammals it is easy to pass a tube into the trachea, with a resultant aspiration pneumonia, when the fluids are given. In tortoises the opening to the trachea is found in the proximal third of the tongue on the floor of the mouth. It is usually clamped tightly shut and so passing the tube into the trachea is very difficult. Keep the lubricated tube dorsal to the tongue by running it along the soft palate into the pharynx (Fig. 9).

Care should be taken whenever large volumes of fluid are to be given by this method. Large amounts of fluid are best passed in several small attempts. This will prevent colic due to overdilation of the intestinal lumen or reflux/passive regurgitation of excessive fluid and secondary aspiration pneumonia. Tortoises should be held upright for a short period after they have been stomach tubed. Care should also be taken not to use too small a diameter catheter. It is possible for these to be bitten through, requiring skilled removal. A gag may be of use in some animals.

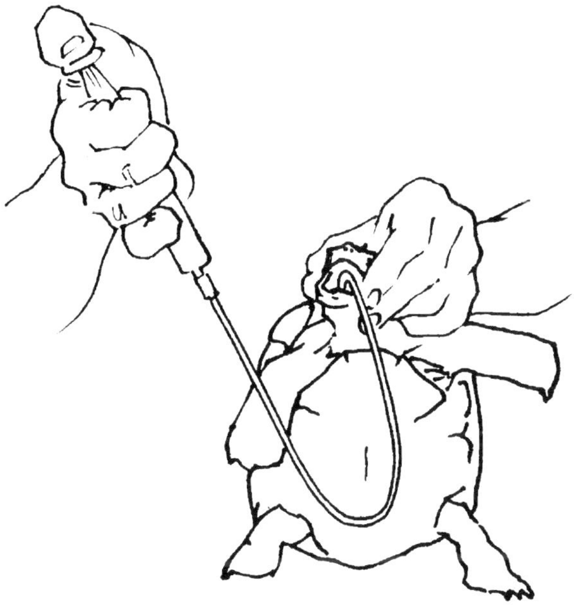

**Fig. 9** Passing a stomach tube. When passing a stomach tube lubricate the end with K-Y jelly (Johnson & Johnson) or similar. If a mouth infection is present then an antibiotic ointment, e.g. neomycin, may be more suitable. The tube is pre-loaded with liquid and run dorsally along the soft palate, this avoids the entrance to the trachea which is located in the proximal third of the tongue. Administer fluids in small amounts, over a suitable period of time, as this will prevent reflux or over dilation of the digestive tract.

## ITEMS TO FORCE FEED

The amount given should never exceed the intake of a healthy tortoise.

| | |
|---|---|
| **Water** | • In renal failure, to flush the kidneys |
| **Rehydration solutions** | • Post-operatively<br>• Pre-operatively<br>• For maintenance during disease<br>• During drug therapy |
| **Vegetable and fruit babyfood preparations** | • For maintenance |
| **Normal tortoise diet in liquidized form** | • For maintenance |

A rough guide is in the region of 1–4% of the animal's body weight expressed in ml spread over a 24-hour period. The amount and frequency of feeding an inactive tortoise would be best decreased from this to prevent stagnation of food. The table below is suitable for an animal such as a temperature-damaged tortoise but food should be offered less frequently in severely debilitated specimens being nursed for long periods of time.

**Table to show suggested volume of food and fluids required in relation to body size for maintenance. These can be decreased if the animal is particularly inactive.** (From Highfield 1992.)

| Body size | Foodstuff | Fluids |
|---|---|---|
| Small tortoise (75–120 mm) | 2 ml twice daily | 5 ml twice daily |
| Medium tortoise (120–180 mm) | 4–5 ml twice daily | 8 ml twice daily |
| Large tortoise (180 mm and more) | 10 ml twice daily | 20–25 ml twice daily |

## SHALLOW BATHING

Shallow bathing a tortoise encourages drinking and urination. Most tortoises find bathing in shallow water that lies just above the level of the

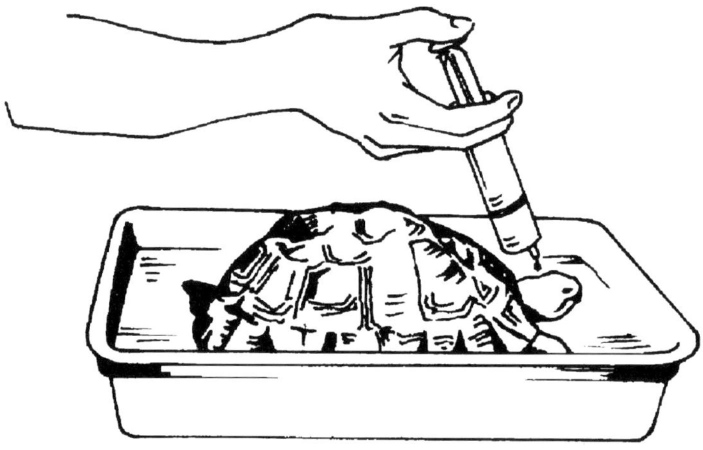

**Fig. 10** Shallow bathing a tortoise encourages drinking and urination.

plastron most pleasurable throughout the year. Some tortoises must immerse their nostrils before their drink. This can look most alarming when seen for the first time.

# HIBERNATION

Mediterranean tortoises have been hibernated with varying success in the UK for several decades. The following information tries to draw together useful information with regard to seeing Mediterranean tortoises through a prolonged winter, in latitudes further north than their countries of origin. Hibernation details for other species are mentioned later, where appropriate, in the section entitled 'The natural environment and husbandry of Chelonia'.

Some authors feel that hibernation of tortoises in northern European latitudes does not seem to serve any necessary purpose and perhaps causes regular problems. Other authors suggest that a short hibernation is important in preventing young animals from growing too quickly and perhaps to allow a shutdown of hormones over winter with a surge when the hibernation finishes. The truth may be a combination of both points of view. It is important to limit, monitor, shorten or even in some situations avoid hibernation. A short and safe hibernation may be completed without problems, but a well planned 'overwintering' where the animal does not hibernate may decrease the number of diseases that are a direct result of hibernation.

Tortoises alter their natural behaviour at the end of the summer in response to falling diurnal temperatures and decreasing daylength. Tortoises stop eating and become less active. It is at this time that a well-managed tortoise should be in optimum condition with ample body fat reserves to see it through the following hibernation period. In hibernating Mediterranean tortoises in northern latitudes we will be exposing these animals to metabolic stresses beyond those they would naturally encounter in the wild. Do not assume these animals are able to look after themselves without careful management.

## HIBERNATION PREPARATION

- Jackson (1985) suggested that the autumn equinox was an important watershed in committing a tortoise to hibernation. He stressed that by this time animals should be divided into those to be hibernated and those to be over wintered so that each can be provided with appropriate husbandry.

- Tortoises should be carefully checked both prior to and after hibernation as a matter of routine.
- Tortoises should never be put into hibernation when they have recently eaten. A pre-hibernation period of four weeks or more without food is recommended for an average-sized animal. Small animals may require less, very large animals somewhat longer. Complications include ear abscessation due to infection ascending the eustachian tube from necrotic food in the buccal cavity. Necrotizing infections, septicaemia and secondary toxin absorption are also possibilities.
- Tortoises should be encouraged to drink prior to hibernation. Some authors suggest that the tortoise may well use the fluid stored within its bladder as its fluid reservoir. Should this fluid reserve be voided it may be unwise to continue hibernation as hydration status may not be maintainable. Tortoises usually urinate after rising only after they have taken fresh fluids on board.
- ***Tortoises that are ill/debilitated, under treatment for a specific illness or are underweight with inadequate fat reserves should not be hibernated.*** Such animals are likely to die during hibernation or awake significantly worse than when they commenced their hibernation.
- It has long been somewhat of a tradition for clients to bring their tortoises to veterinary surgeons for a prehibernation vitamin injection. Whilst this procedure is unlikely to do harm, it should not be required in a well-managed animal that has received appropriate supplementation throughout the season. Injection site abscesses, irritation and overdose are possible complications. It is far more important for the veterinary surgeon to perform a full clinical examination in order to help the client decide whether or not to hibernate the tortoise.

**A summary of pre-hibernation preparations**

- Check the tortoise's health early in the autumn (before the equinox).
- Check the tortoise's weight routinely but especially at the start of hibernation.
- Ensure the tortoise has not eaten within four weeks of hibernation.
- Confirm that the tortoise has been provided with the opportunity to drink before hibernation.
- Ensure hibernation facilities offer protection from extreme temperature changes, are well-ventilated, are away from car fumes, are checked regularly throughout the hibernation for suitable temperature range and are secure from dangers such as rodent attack.

## WEIGHT AND LENGTH MEASUREMENTS IN RELATION TO HIBERNATION

Tortoises should be weighed and measured, as suggested by Jackson (1980b; 1985) and subsequent authors, at regular intervals throughout the year (see Fig. 4).

| | |
|---|---|
| **Weight** | • Should be measured in grams (g) |
| **Straight carapace length (SCL)** | • Should be measured in millimetres (mm) |

## THE INTERPRETATION OF WEIGHT/LENGTH MEASUREMENTS

It is important to encourage clients to regularly monitor their animal's weight. Failure to accumulate adequate body fat and reach a suitable pre-hibernation weight implies ill health or poor husbandry that will require suitable investigation.

The graph of weight and length measurements produced by Jackson (1980b) in the early eighties is included with kind permission of the BSAVA (Fig. 11). This graph is often used to assess health and the suitability of hibernation. However, it is important to realize that the data only concerns Mediterranean species and that it will not be accurate to assess other species using this graph. It is wise to plot a Mediterranean tortoise's position on this graph during any clinical examination, however care should be taken in drawing conclusions from this graph alone.

I have also included graphical information of two groups of recently examined Mediterranean tortoises. The first group consists of weight and length measurements of 33 Mediterranean tortoises examined by myself between 1992 and 1994 because of a variety of diseases (Fig. 12). All of the tortoises were ill in some way.

The second group also consists of 33 Mediterranean tortoises owned by members of The Tortoise Trust (Fig. 13). All of this group were healthy. It was not possible to see any significant relationship between health and weight/length data.

The data for both groups was very similar (Fig. 14) and both groups tended to weigh more than was suggested by Jackson (1980b). No animals were recorded as underweight and this would probably reflect the high standards of husbandry practised by UK tortoise owners in order

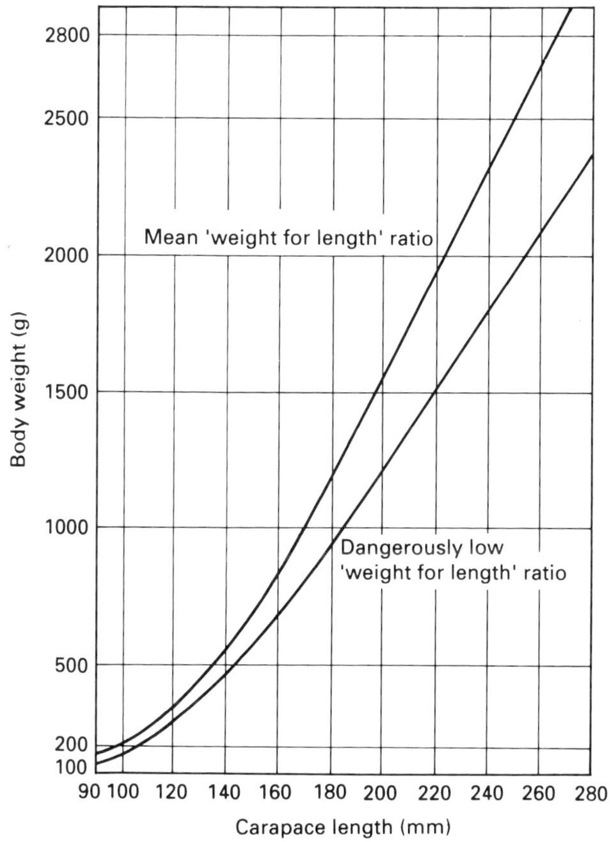


**Fig. 11** Growth of healthy *Testudo graeca* and *Testudo hermanni* in the UK, plotting mass against length (known as the Jackson Ratio). (Reproduced with kind permission of the BSAVA.)

for their pets to have survived so long since importation. Jackson's data included recently imported tortoises which are no longer seen.

- Animals suffering from chronic illness may retain fluid and be significantly overweight. Any significantly overweight animal should be examined closely for renal and hepatic problems. Hibernation should not be attempted if illness is suspected.
- A tortoise may be assumed to lose 1% of its body weight during each month of hibernation. Hibernation periods in this country may easily reach 20 or more weeks if animals are left unmanaged. Smaller tortoises should be observed closely as they have proportionately less fat reserves. It is therefore important to restrict the duration of hibernation for these animals.

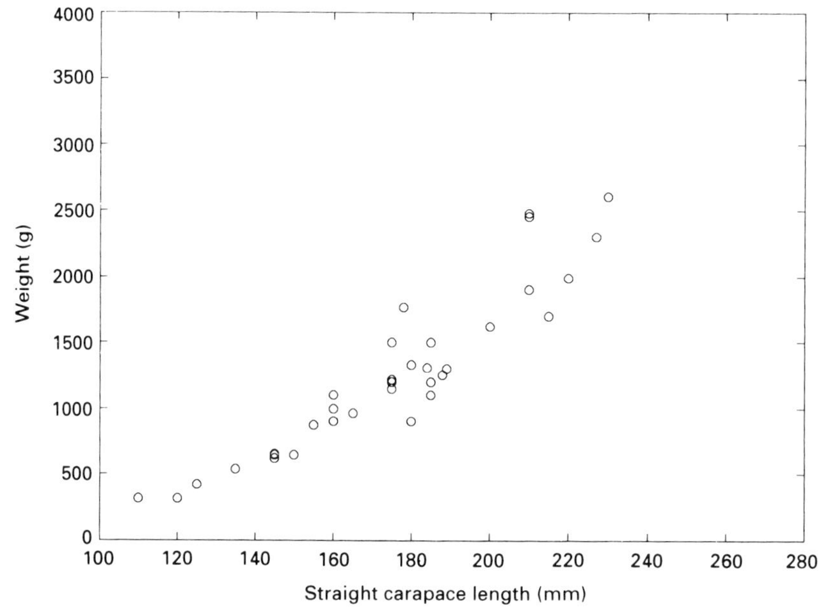


**Fig. 12** Weight:SCL relationships of ill Mediterranean tortoises 1992–4.

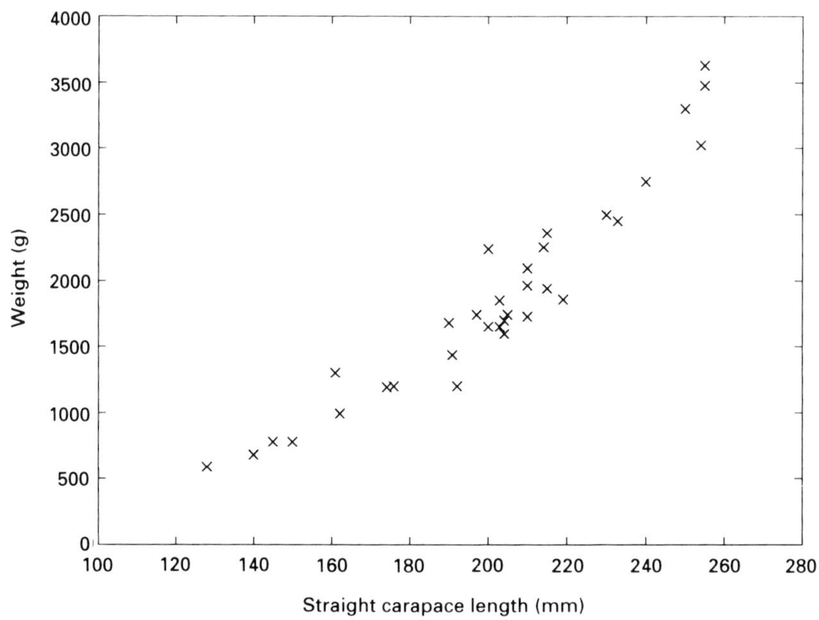


**Fig. 13** Weight:SCL relationships of healthy Mediterranean tortoises summer 1992.

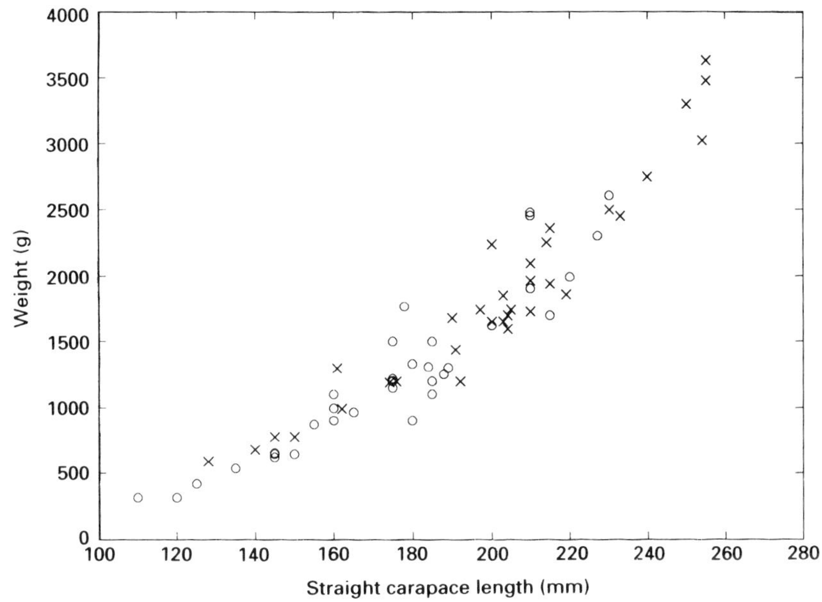


**Fig. 14** Weight:SCL relationships of both groups combined.

- Post-hibernation weights are also of value. A tortoise that attempts to continue hibernation in too warm an environment (at or above 10°C) will have a raised metabolic rate compared to a tortoise hibernating at 5°C, consequently it will exhaust its fat reserves early and build up high concentrations of metabolic toxins, as protein catabolism occurs. Weight loss above that expected for a normal hibernation implies that hibernation duration and temperature may not have been ideal. Such animals must be managed carefully in order to deal with any post-hibernation problems that may occur. This is particularly important in winters when warm spells occur early and are then followed by cold spells whilst hibernation has not yet finished.

## IDEAL CONDITIONS DURING HIBERNATION (see Fig. 15)

### Temperature

- Hibernation is significantly temperature dependent although photoperiodic reduction also plays a part. It is precipitated by the ambient daytime temperatures falling below 10°C.
- The optimal maintenance temperature throughout hibernation is about 5°C. Temperatures below 2°C are potentially dangerous, and at temperatures above about 11°C tortoises tend to become active.

- At sub-zero temperatures sight damage or brain damage may occur. Even short-term exposure can result in long-term and permanent injury. This problem is common in tortoises hibernated out of doors, in garden sheds or garages, without adequate protection. It is important to note that a large number of patients who present as 'not feeding' following hibernation will, on further investigation, prove to have suffered frost damage. Certainly, any tortoise which is moving in circles, failing to respond adequately to visual stimuli and is reported as 'anorexic' should be regarded as a probable frost-damage case.
- Apparently some UK tortoise owners are now using carefully monitored fridges for hibernation. A daily check ensures an air change and temperatures can be accurately maintained.

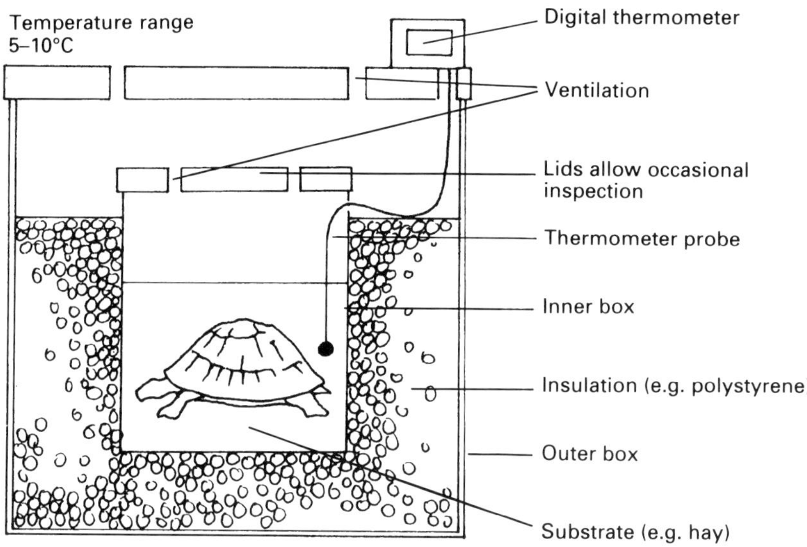


**Fig. 15** A cross-section of suitable hibernation facilities for the Mediterranean tortoise.

## Duration of hibernation

| **Influences on the duration of hibernation include** |
| --- |
| • Weather<br>• Latitude<br>• Fat reserves<br>• Species<br>• Size and age<br>• Health status |

- The autumn equinox is considered to be the time at which animals commit themselves to hibernation. If a tortoise requires over-wintering then it is best to provide artificial heat and light from this time onwards so that the metabolism does not wind down towards hibernation status.
- In England hibernation usually starts in October/November. The further north the location, the earlier tortoises tend to be ready for hibernation. If left unmanaged hibernation may finish about April. The duration may therefore be five or six months. This is far longer than would occur in a natural environment and this is reflected in the frequency of post-hibernation problems encountered in this country.
- Tortoise owners should be encouraged to manage the duration and seasonal timing of their animal's hibernation. The provision of a 'synthetically prolonged autumn' and a 'synthetically early spring' in order to maintain a short, safe hibernation is wise.
- A hibernation period should not exceed 20 weeks. In a more natural latitude it may be as short as 4–6 weeks. Hibernation is not essential. It can be avoided with appropriate husbandry.

### Continued management

Hibernating tortoises can be handled and checked quite safely. Many owners believe that handling a hibernating tortoise is ill-advised, but in fact the opposite is true. Regular checks can be a life-safer.

- It would be advisable to wake a tortoise if the hibernation is not proceeding as expected due to ill health (e.g. skin/shell disease, trauma, etc.). The remainder of the expected hibernation period can be as described for overwintering tortoises.
- It is not advisable to continue hibernation if spontaneous urination is detected. Such animals should be woken to prevent dehydration.
- Upon awakening tortoises should be encouraged to drink as soon as possible. This may be assisted by bathing in shallow water.
- If a tortoise wakes and eats, during an early spring warm spell, do not let it hibernate if it gets cold again.

## OVERWINTERING TORTOISES

Tortoises can be overwintered, this is the prevention of hibernation by provision of a suitable environment for the tortoise to remain awake throughout the winter. These tortoises should be supplemented with both light and heat from autumn onwards.

The optimal temperature range of overwintered Mediterranean tortoises is 18–25°C during daytime, falling to 14–16°C during the night. Humidity can be maintained by the provision of pots of gravel in the vivaria which can be kept slightly damp to produce evaporation. Many overwintered tortoises suffer from dry eyes and skin if inadequate levels of humidity are provided (Fig. 16).

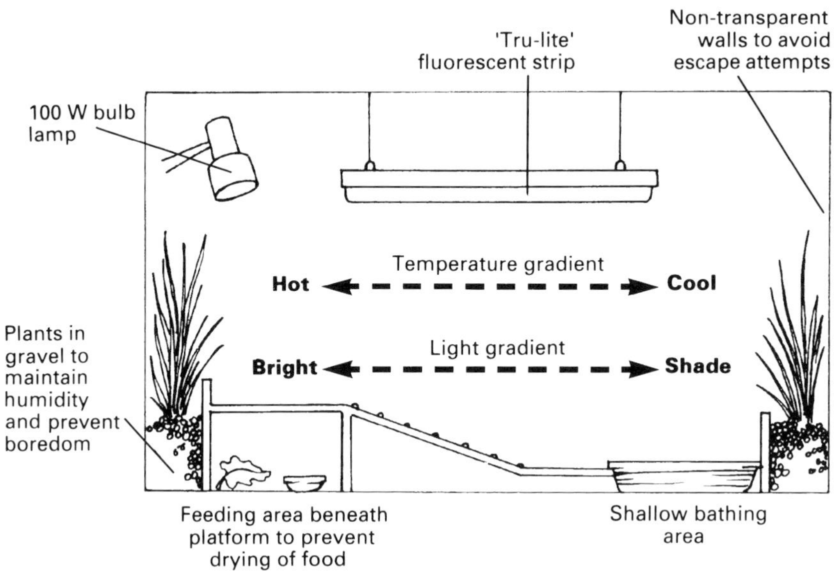


**Fig. 16** A suitable area in which a Mediterranean tortoise may be overwintered.

- Most tortoises require very bright illumination in order to stimulate feeding. 'Tru-lite' tubes are desirable as they may allow continued activation of vitamin $D_3$. Incandescent bulbs of 100–150 W will suffice if adequate vitamin D is otherwise available. Multiple bulbs are often required.
- Heat can be provided using a ceramic infrared heat bulb in a screw-in socket, thermotubes, or heat pads. Incandescent spotlights are also useful. The clip-on types allow greater freedom of choice with respect of placement.
- A temperature and light gradient is advised. This allows the tortoise the ability to move from the bright warm area to a cooler shaded area as it desires, and hence to thermoregulate naturally.
- Food should normally be provided at the brighter end of the accommodation, but should not be situated directly under heat sources (to prevent drying).

- It is very important that overwintering tortoises should be provided with regular baths to encourage drinking and prevent dehydration.

A conservatory or adequately heated greenhouse with natural daylight is a considerable asset and can quickly be converted into a first-rate terrarium. Light will still require supplementation in order to provide an adequate daylength for feeding. As glass will filter UV light, it would still be wise to ensure vitamin $D_3$ activation is able to occur. Vitamin supplementation would be wise.

## POST-HIBERNATION PHYSIOLOGICAL CHANGES

The low metabolic rate during hibernation and the maintenance of a prolonged period of inactivity results in many physiological changes upon awakening.

**A tortoise that has recently hibernated will have**

- Low fat reserves
- A low white blood cell count
- A poor level of hydration
- Accumulated high levels of metabolic toxins (e.g. urea/urates)
- An increased level of protein catabolism to provide energy
- A low blood glucose level and little glycogen reserves
- Low levels of vitamins, especially those fat soluble

(Lawrence 1987; Lawrence & Jackson 1983a)

**The following conditions are often apparent in the post-hibernation period**

- Eye, nerve and brain damage as a result of exposure to excessively low temperatures
- Mouth infections (necrotic stomatitis)
- Upper respiratory infections (runny nose syndrome)
- Shell damage from rodent attack
- Chronic debility (e.g. vitamin A deficiency)
- Jaundice
- Post-hibernation anorexia (PHA)

## A POST-HIBERNATION CLINICAL EXAMINATION

- Compare weight measurements to pre-hibernation values.
- Compare weight measurements to species averages.

- Use regular weight measurements to assess progress throughout the season.

Blood urea levels are at their highest in the immediate post-hibernation period. This is due to the combination of a build-up of metabolic toxins and dehydration. If the weather has been too mild during the late hibernation period, or fat reserves have been inadequate, protein catabolism to supply energy will have begun. This will further add to blood urea levels. Lawrence (1987) pointed out that blood urea levels approaching 200 mmol/litre are consistently fatal in the post-hibernation period. The implication was that urate levels are also high and precipitation of urate within the renal tubules resulted in kidney failure as did the nephrotoxic effect of metabolites.

***Animals with blood urea levels approaching 150 mmol/litre can sometimes be saved by appropriate fluid therapy.***

It is vital that tortoises drink within 24–48 hours of emergence. This can be assisted by shallow bathing the tortoise in a bath of water, about 2 cm deep for an average animal. This tends to cause simultaneous drinking and urination, flushing urea and other toxins out. Many tortoise owners have observed that their animal will only urinate after it has drunk. Any animal that has not drunk within this time period should be administered fluids, by stomach tube if required. The nature of the fluid is debatable but as urination is the desired aim, a plain water solution would seem appropriate. Later, fluids can be altered to promote retention in body tissue as with traditional rehydration solutions. Lawrence (1987) discussed the fact that renal function is absent when plasma osmolarity rises above about 100 mosm/litre. Diluting the blood concentration is therefore a primary aim.

## ASSESS NUTRITION

Most healthy animals eat within one week of emergence from hibernation. Lawrence (1987) stated that animals that had not eaten within seven weeks of rising, with or without treatment, should be given a very poor prognosis. Most animals favour succulent foods with a high moisture content immediately post-hibernation (e.g. cucumber, tomatoes and fruits) but should be offered a more balanced diet within a few days. Lawrence (1987) indicated that blood glucose levels have a significant effect on appetite. A peak blood glucose level is produced in healthy animals within the first few days of rising but animals who do not eat within this time and so do not maintain blood glucose levels, or animals unable to release sufficient levels of glucose into the bloodstream, are likely to remain anorexic for some time if appropriate treatment is not given. Failure to eat within a reasonable time of rising from hibernation is termed post-hibernation anorexia (PHA). Suggestions as to how PHA can be dealt with are given in the next section 'Post-hibernation anorexia'.

## ASSESS ENVIRONMENT

Tortoises require good climatic conditions in order to thrive. It is always wise to compare their captive environment to a typical natural one and to try and mimic these conditions as closely as possible. Grey, dull, cold miserable springs result in prolonged inappetence. The least one should do is to offer protection and shelter in the evenings and at night.

**It is advisable to supplement**

- Duration of daylight
- Temperature
- Humidity
- Light intensity

# POST-HIBERNATION ANOREXIA (PHA)

Post-hibernation anorexia (PHA) is perhaps one of the most likely reasons for presentation of a tortoise at the veterinary surgery in the immediate post-hibernation period. PHA encompasses anorexia in the early season for a variety of reasons. These may be physiological, pathological or environmental. It has been well examined by Lawrence (1987), Lawrence & Jackson (1983a), Jackson (1985) and Highfield (1986). Post-hibernation anorexia is the term used to describe animals that fail to eat within an acceptable period of rising from hibernation. Highfield (1992) states that in dealing with a large number of healthy tortoises, most eat within 24 to 48 hours of rising. Lawrence (1987) stated figures of ten days without drinking and three to four weeks without eating as requiring treatment. The earlier an intervention is achieved for an animal with PHA, the better will be the consequent prognosis. Lawrence (1987) also stated that should the period of anorexia rise to seven weeks then it is an indication for giving a guarded prognosis. PHA carries a varying prognosis depending on the underlying condition of the animal and the delay in achieving treatment.

The reasons for PHA are complex and in need of continued research. To keep things simple the veterinary surgeon should consider the following classification:

- **Complicated PHA** (pathological).

Here clinical examination reveals concomitant disease that in itself may result in anorexia. Necrotic stomatitis and runny nose syndrome are such diseases but eye damage due to exposure to excessively cold temperatures and the summation of chronic debility and malnutrition over the past seasons are also common.

- **Uncomplicated PHA** (physiological or environmental).

This is not so common in my experience. Such animals are likely to be suffering from a physiological or metabolic problem such as dehydration, uraemia, low blood glucose levels or any combination of these. This is often due to unsuitable hibernation or an excessively long, poorly prepared or badly managed hibernation. It may be that the problem relates to poor post-hibernation management. Heat, light and humidity are important in the stimulation of appetite and should be monitored closely and supplemented as required in the critical post-hibernation period.

## HISTORY

**This should include the following details from the client**

- Progress made in previous years.
- Environment and climatic conditions.
- The condition of other tortoises owned by the client.
- The quality of husbandry.
- The quality of nutrition provided by the client.
- The degree of health checks performed by the client and their frequency throughout the year.

## CLINICAL EXAMINATION

The veterinary surgeon should identify the case as being complicated or uncomplicated. Complicated cases will require specific treatment and management relating to the underlying pathology. This should be carried out in parallel to treatment one would provide for any uncomplicated PHA animal. Lawrence (1987) investigated cases of uncomplicated PHA and drew the following conclusions:

**Cases of uncomplicated PHA**

- Animals usually have a lower than expected weight to length ratio.
- They tend to be dehydrated and have an elevated packed cell volume (PCV).
- They tend to have a very low blood glucose level <5 mmol/litre.
- They have elevated blood urea levels (about 200 mmol/litre being fatal but 150 mmol/litre responding to rapid appropriate treatment).
- The *BSAVA Manual of Reptiles* (1992) also points out that PHA cases are often presented with a jaundice that responds to appropriate PHA management in non-severe cases.

## TREATMENT

**The primary aims of treatment should be**

- To correct dehydration.
- To achieve diuresis and consequently decrease the elevated blood urea levels, flushing lethal toxins through the kidneys.
- To elevate the blood glucose levels.
- To provide optimal environmental conditions.
- To treat any underlying disease or nutritional disorder effectively.
- To provide nutrition by handfeeding or via stomach tube feeding. As described in the text concerning forced feeding, in the section on 'Handling, injection and feeding techniques'.

## TREATMENT ADVICE

- Administer fluids by stomach tube. A parenteral route can also be used in severe debility.
- The nature of the fluid will vary with the effect desired. The initial uraemic presentation will first require hypotonic fluids such as water. This will promote diuresis and the voiding of toxins and will decrease plasma osmolarity, restoring renal function.
- Having achieved renal function, blood glucose levels should be assessed. It is suggested that blood glucose levels show a temporary surge in the normal post-hibernation period. If a tortoise fails to produce such a surge or fails to maintain this level long enough to eat, then this in itself will result in anorexia. It is glucose solutions that are required next. It has been suggested that Liquid Lectade (SmithKline Beecham) is appropriate as it will produce a blood glucose surge comparable to that seen in ruminants with low blood sugar levels (e.g. twin lamb disease) and depending on the dilution used will help address dehydration (A. Routh, personal communication). Other solutions suggested include traditional rehydration sachets and Hartmann's solution or saline with glucose.
- These glucose solutions can then be supplemented with appropriate nutrition. This should include solutions of vitamins (e.g. Abidec: W-L, Nutrobal: Vetark Professional, ACE-High: Vetark Professional, Vionate: Sherleys) and liquidized food appropriate to the normal animal diet. A blender or food processor will help here. Baby foods with appropriate constituents can also be used. There is some circumstantial evidence to suggest that the lactose content of Complan is not appropriate to the herbivorous tortoise's digestive system. It

would perhaps be wise to avoid such solutions until this has been investigated further.

- As a response is produced the handler should transfer to syringe and hand feeding techniques as soon as possible. It should be the aim to feed normal dietary constituents as soon as is feasible.
- Concurrent disease must be investigated and appropriately treated.
- Appropriate environmental temperatures, humidity, and light intensity should be provided. A cold, dry tortoise in a dark cat kennel cannot be expected to achieve activity and self-nutrition.

# NUTRITION

Most commonly encountered Mediterranean tortoises are herbivorous, but the dietary requirements of omnivorous tortoises, such as the African hingeback and the American box turtle, are also mentioned.

## FOODS FOR HERBIVOROUS TORTOISES

Cat or dog food, bread and milk (substances which are occasionally recommended in some pet care publications) are contraindicated for inclusion in the dietary regime of *herbivorous* tortoises. Renal and hepatic problems commonly result following long term consumption. Milk-based nutritional compounds such as Complan are also questionable on the grounds that some tortoises appear to demonstrate severe gastric side effects, possibly as a result of lactose intolerance. Such foods are also inadequate in fibre content. Earlier texts used these products with apparently good results but current thinking is starting to feel these may be unsuitable. Hand feeding programmes should instead rely upon liquidized natural-type foods.

A diet should be:

- **low** in fats, oils and proteins
- **rich** in minerals and vitamins
- **high** in fibre
- **adequate** in water content.

The following dietary components are suggested for:

- *Testudo hermanni*
- *Testudo horsfieldi*
- *Testudo marginata*
- *Testudo graeca*.

| Mixed green-leaf vegetable base | Fruits and succulents |
|---|---|
| • Dandelion leaves | • Melon |
| • Cabbage (mixed varieties) | • Tomato |
| • Clover shoots | • Mango |
| • Kale parsley | • Cauliflower |
| • Carrot tops | • Apple |
| • Sowthistle | • Pear |
| • Mixed grasses | • Peppers |
| • Chickweed | • Cucumber |
| | • Marrow |

Daily supplementation with a suitable vitamin and mineral preparation is advised at all times (e.g. Vionate: Sherleys).

Fruits should be fed cautiously in animals with digestive disturbances as the high sugar levels can encourage bacterial and protozoal overgrowth. This is particularly important after antibiotic treatments.

## PREPARATION OF FOOD

Tortoises are well known for having very capricious appetites. It is advisable to offer food in mixtures blended together. A food processor is useful here. The various ingredients can be mixed together with a vitamin supplement and offered fresh daily as a sort of raw coleslaw. Mixing food avoids malnutrition and addiction to a narrow base of limited value foods.

## FOODS FOR OMNIVOROUS TORTOISES AND TURTLES

### THE BOX TURTLE (*Terrapene* spp.)

Young *Terrapene* spp. are particularly carnivorous but as they mature the tendency is for a higher proportion of vegetable matter to be consumed.

| Hatchlings feed almost exclusively on small prey such as | Mature animals will also require fruit and vegetables such as |
|---|---|
| • Earthworms | • Banana |
| • Slugs | • Mushroom |
| • Pupae | • Apple |
| • Maggots | • Pears |

A daily vitamin supplement, such as Nutrobal: Vetark Professional, Vionate: Sherleys or ACE-High: Vetark Professional, is advised and a small amount of meat, fish or low fat dog food may be offered occasionally. The fat content of some cat and dog foods is particularly high and these should be avoided. Again a balanced and varied diet is better than an addiction to a limited variety of foods.

## THE AFRICAN HINGEBACK (*Kinyxis* spp.)

African hingebacks are omnivorous and insectivorous.

**Preferred diet of African hingebacks includes**

- Snails
- Millipedes
- Fallen fruit
- Grasses
- General vegetation
- Mushrooms
- Lettuce
- Bananas
- Tomatoes
- Peaches

A small amount of low-fat dog food can be offered occasionally, about once a week is suggested.

A calcium rich supplement such as Nutrobal: Vetark Professional is advised on a regular basis.

## THE RED-EARED TERRAPIN (*Pseudemys scripta elegans*) AND THE EUROPEAN POND TURTLE (*Emrys orbicularis*)

These terrapins are omnivorous and thrive on both animal and plant material in suitable combinations. Commercial turtle flakes tend to be lacking in minerals and vitamins whilst feeding oily fish in large quantities may result in steatitis/fatty liver and B vitamin deficiency due to excess of thiaminases. A suitable diet will consist of a range of products that complement each other.

**Suitable dietary constituents for freshwater turtles**

- Turtle flakes
- Plant leaf material
- Fruits
- Canned dog food
- Raw whole fish
- Rehydrated cat or dog pellets
- Pond fish pellets
- Insects
- Fresh meat (liver)

Rehydrated foods will benefit from additional supplementation with mineral/vitamin preparations and ACE-High: Vetark Professional, Vionate: Sherleys, Nutrobal: Vetark Professional are all suitable.

Diets that centre around animal protein tend to have a high phosphorus level in relation to calcium; this may well result in abnormal shell and bone growth. Supplementation with some accessible form of calcium, such as Nutrobal: Vetark Professional will counteract this as will offering cuttlefish bone to be gnawed.

**Water filtration**

Maintaining good water quality is essential as the incidence of bacterial and parasitic diseases will increase rapidly when this is not attended. A motorized filtration system is essential, as are regular water changes.

# SPECIFIC NUTRITIONAL DISORDERS

These are relatively common in tortoises owned by clients who have fed diets with no supplementation of vitamins and that have been to the preference of the animal rather than a diet from a reputable text.

| Common conditions include |
|---|
| • Vitamin A deficiency<br>• Vitamin $D_3$ deficiency and nutritional osteodystrophy<br>• Visceral and articular gout<br>• Iodine deficiency<br>• Steatitis<br>• Renal failure<br>• Hepatic failure |

## VITAMIN A DEFICIENCY

Vitamin A is fat soluble and consequently tends to be low, or even absent, in many client fed diets. Having poor fat reserves means that tortoises require a constant low level intake of vitamin A in order to avoid deficiencies. Vitamin A deficiency tends to be a problem seen after a deficient diet has been fed for some time. A tortoise presented with clinical signs may have suffered the nutritional insult the year before. The role of vitamin A is in the production of healthy epithelia. Deficiency can manifest in many ways and may be picked up when the diet of an animal assumed to be suffering from another disease such as runny nose syndrome is examined. Because of its essential role in maintaining health in the tortoise it is recommended that all animals are constantly supplemented with a low level of vitamin A.

Deficiency results in metaplasia and degeneration of epithelial surfaces such as conjunctiva, gingiva, pancreatic ducts, renal tubules, skin and lung alveoli.

Vitamin A deficiency is relatively common in the common terrapin (*Pseudemys scripta elegans*). This usually responds well to supplementation with a vitamin supplement and the inclusion of vitamin A rich food such as liver.

| Signs of vitamin A deficiency |
|---|
| • Swollen eyes/conjunctivitis<br>• Skin sloughing<br>• Runny nose syndrome<br>• Necrotic stomatitis<br>• Respiratory problems<br>• Jaundice/renal failure/death |

**Treatment**

- Prevention of nutritional disease is better than cure. ***Regular supplementation with a vitamin–mineral additive, such as Vionate: Sherleys or ACE-High: Vetark Professional, is highly recommended for all tortoises and turtles.*** Examine the normal diet for any possible deficiencies or unsuitable components.
- Any secondary condition should be treated suitably, e.g. gentamicin cream or ointment to protect damaged skin.
- The practice of a pre-hibernation vitamin A injection fails to address any underlying nutritional problem and, as it is not significantly stored, it is of extremely limited therapeutic value.

## VITAMIN A TOXICITY

Vitamin A toxicity manifests in a very similar fashion to deficiency with skin and conjunctival hyperplasia and skin sloughing. It can occur as a result of overdosing a primary source of vitamin A that requires no activation within the body, e.g. vitamin A injections. It is far better to address the diet of the animal suspected of a vitamin A deficiency than to actively inject it with large doses of vitamin A. The dosage of vitamin A therapy included later in the drug tables should not be administered more than once a week. Repeated doses should not be required if any inappropriate diet has been corrected (Zwart 1987).

## VITAMIN $D_3$ DEFICIENCY AND NUTRITIONAL OSTEODYSTROPHY

These conditions have been described by many authors including Highfield (1990), Cooper (1985), Jackson & Fasal (1981), Jackson (1980a) and Keymer (1978a; 1978b). They occur in both aquatic carnivorous Chelonia and herbivorous terrestrial tortoises. They are the result of unsuitable mineral and vitamin content in the diet.

The following have been suggested as predisposing factors:

- feeding a diet without any mineral or vitamin supplementation (e.g. lettuce only);
- feeding a high protein diet, particularly if low in calcium;
- use of unsuitable artificial light source, decreasing vitamin $D_3$ activation.

The ideal ratio of calcium to phosphorus in the diet is often suggested to be in the range 4:1 or 6:1.

As most green vegetation has a high level of phosphate it is wise to consider the addition of a calcium-rich supplement such as Nutrobal: Vetark Professional. This could also be mixed with Vionate: Sherleys to provide an excellent all round supplement with adequate vitamin $D_3$ and calcium. Vionate: Sherleys on its own is not particularly rich in calcium. Offering cuttlefish can also be beneficial.

## Diagnosis

The signs of nutritional osteodystrophy differ between terrapins and tortoises. The signs are more exaggerated if the nutritional imbalance is present at the time when growth is occurring.

In tortoises, abnormal growth of the carapace is apparent and the scutes tend to change in angle resulting in so called 'pyramiding'. The shell often appears undersized compared to the limbs and head. Other findings reported include a softening of the plastron, leg weakness and deformity. Young herbivorous animals can sometimes produce rapid and excessive growth when fed on abnormally high levels of protein. First impressions are of high growth rate and good husbandry but this soon changes when obvious and irreversible deformities of the skeletal system arise. It is unwise to offer high protein diets (meat, dog food, etc.) to increase growth rates. Books such as Highfield (1990) discuss juvenile diets in detail.

In the terrapin the main findings are 'soft-shell'. Here the animal's shell is weakened to the extent that it is relatively easily compressed by finger pressure (see Plate 5).

Jackson & Fasal (1981) describe the radiographic changes apparent with this condition as decreased radio density of bony tissues such as the pelvis and limbs, sometimes to the extent that the animal is difficult

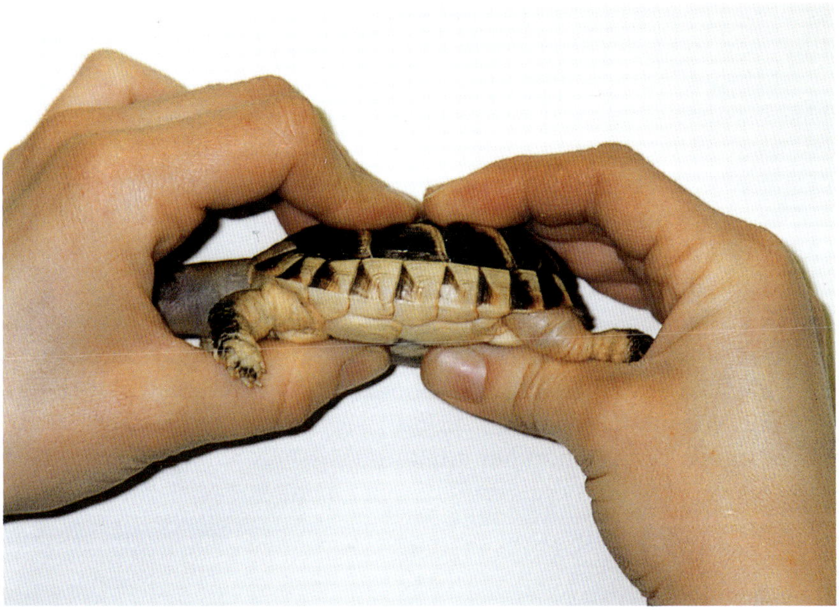

**Plate 5** Soft shell or secondary nutrition osteodystrophy in a one-year-old spur thighed tortoise. This case is the result of an unsuitably high protein diet without mineral or vitamin supplementation. The plastron and carapace of this moribund tortoise were easily depressed with light digit pressure. The bloated, oedematous skin demonstrates fluid retention during renal failure. A lack of pigmentation, abnormally large size and soft disproportionate limbs were also apparent.

to radiograph. They also advise the close examination of the 'pillars' or axiliary/inguinal scutes for radiolucency.

Fowler (1986) points out that feeding excessive amounts of dog or cat foods with high vitamin D can result in the opposite situation of heavy, and perhaps even fatal, soft tissue mineralization. Great care should be taken when offering these products to reptiles.

### Treatment

- Correct dietary problems.
- Correct environmental problems.
- Vitamin $D_3$ by injection (take care not to overdose).

## VISCERAL AND ARTICULAR GOUT

Where renal function is impaired, or renal excretion of urates is inadequate, the blood levels of uric acid and urates rise. If the blood level of these substances reaches a sufficient level then urate compounds crystallize and so are deposited in tissues, this is termed gout. In the tortoise these tissues can be intrarenal/pericardial (visceral) or in the joint spaces of distal limbs (articular). Crystallization and deposition of urates will result in damage to the affected area. If this is renal, then the problem can be self-perpetuating and possibly even fatal.

There is circumstantial evidence to suggest an increased incidence of gout where diets with excessive protein are being fed. Similarly, long-term dehydration may have an exacerbating effect. Animals with long standing vitamin A deficiencies may also end up with secondary gout due to renal dysfunction. This is as a result of epithelial metaplasia of the renal tubules and resulting decreased renal excretion of urates. The red-eared terrapin (*Pseudemys scripta elegans*) is particularly prone to this. Animals receiving nephrotoxic drugs, such as aminoglycosides, may also develop gout as a result of renal damage.

### Diagnosis

- Diagnosis of gout in Chelonia is usually retrospective.
- Visceral gout can be seen radiographically as an increased opacity or mineralization of the organ or tissue concerned (e.g. kidneys). This is often an incidental finding.
- The possibility of urate deposition due to post-hibernation dehydration and metabolic toxin build-up should always be considered in the immediate post-hibernation period. Fluid therapy to restore renal function is discussed later in this section under the heading 'Renal failure'.
- Where facilities are available, blood urea and urate levels will help indicate if gout is likely to be occurring.
- Animals with joint or limb swellings should be investigated for the possibility of gout. Radiography and blood biochemistry will help.

### Treatment

Treatment is unlikely to cause resolution of symptoms. Fluid therapy and attention to nutritional problems may help. Colleagues from the southern hemisphere have suggested that allopurinol (Zyloric: Wellcome), a urease inhibitor, may be of use in reptiles in general, 20 mg/kg has been suggested but there is no information regarding its efficacy. Another suggestion has been to dissolve a 100 mg tablet in 5 ml of water and then offering 1 ml/kg daily by stomach tube.

## IODINE DEFICIENCY

This can result from a diet lacking in iodine where water iodine levels are low, or where goitrogenic substances are fed in excess (e.g. kale, cabbage or sprouts).

**Symptoms include**

- Lethargy or debility
- Oedema
- Goitre
- It has been suggested that T4 blood levels <10 mmol/litre are suggestive of hypothyroidism from this or another cause

### Treatment

- Examine suitability of diet including access to and content of drinking water.
- Supplement the diet as required. Vionate: Sherleys provides 30 mg/kg of iodine and prevents deficiency as do most suitable supplements.
- Thyroxine (e.g. Soloxine: Daniels Pharmaceuticals 0.2 mg every 48 hours orally) has been suggested.

## STEATITIS

This occurs where an excessively fat rich, or otherwise unsuitable diet has been provided, e.g. meat-based dog food, cat food, fish, cheese and dairy products. It has already been pointed out that these foodstuffs are not suited to herbivorous species and should be used carefully, if at all, in omnivorous and carnivorous species.

### Symptoms

- Obesity.
- Nodular fat deposition.
- Fatty liver/jaundice/hepatitis.

### Treatment

Suggested treatments include:

- Injections of anabolic steroids (e.g. Nandrolin: Intervet at 0.5 mg/tortoise weekly).

- Vitamin E as an antioxidant.
- Thyroxine (e.g. Soloxine: Daniels Pharmaceuticals at 0.2 mg/tortoise every 48 hours orally).

## HEPATITIS

As mentioned this occurs with vitamin A deficiency and steatitis. It can also be through infectious disease. Jaundice has been nursed by oral dosing methionine at 250 mg/tortoise every 48 hours for five doses and supportive fluid therapy, but the prognosis is poor if a response is not seen early.

## RENAL FAILURE

Abnormally high protein diets, and other unsuitable unbalanced diets, regularly result in high blood urea and urate levels and fluid retention. This may precipitate and exacerbate renal failure. Tortoises in renal failure tend to present as anorexic and bloated with fluid. Their Jackson ratio calculation tends to present them as particularly heavy. Treatment is often futile. Fluid therapy, anabolic steroids, vitamins and diuretics have been employed, but with limited success. Blood urea and urate levels can be used to monitor renal function, particularly in the critical post-hibernation period. This is discussed under the heading 'Post-hibernation physiological changes' in the section on 'Hibernation' and in the section on 'Laboratory tests and suitable samples'.

## PROTEIN EXCESSES DURING GROWTH

Young tortoises fed on unsuitable high protein diets such as beans or meat often demonstrate remarkable growth rates. This unfortunately tends to culminate in abnormal shell growth with 'soft shell', pyramiding of the scutes and disproportionate limbs and shell size. It is not unusual for extreme cases to present with a light pigmentation of the shell. Terminal renal failure often hinders treatment attempts. See Plates 6 and 7, Figs 17 and 18.

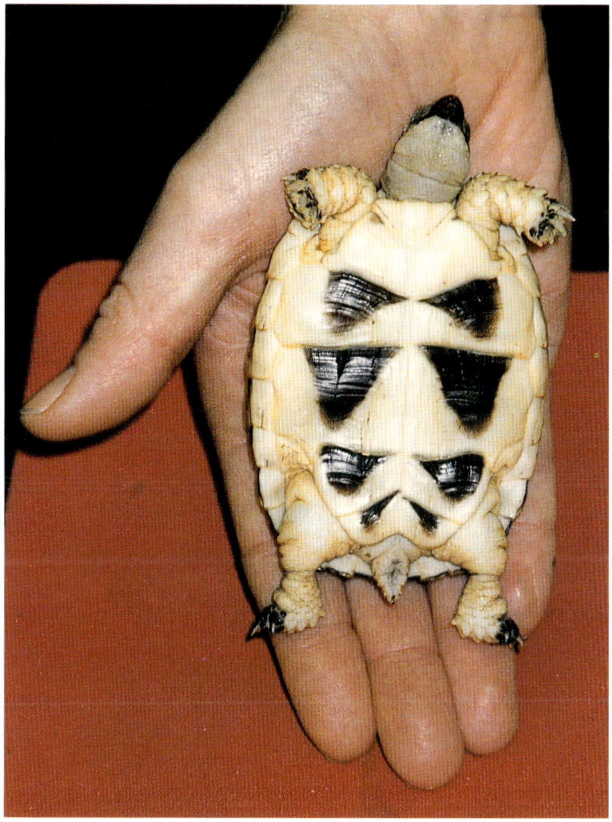

**Plate 6** The effects of an unsuitable high protein diet during periods of growth and development are often irreversible. This one year old North African spur-thighed tortoise (*T. graeca* spp) was fed exclusively on baked beans after its illegal entry to the UK in 1994. It was 2–3 times larger than we had expected. The carapace accounted for the majority of this animal's size and the shell was easily depressed with gentle finger pressure, because of nutritional osteodystrophy (soft shell). The hind limbs were not in proportion to the body size and were particularly fragile. The skin of the sublumbar fossa and neck and shoulders was bloated from fluid retention due to renal failure. This tortoise was euthanased.

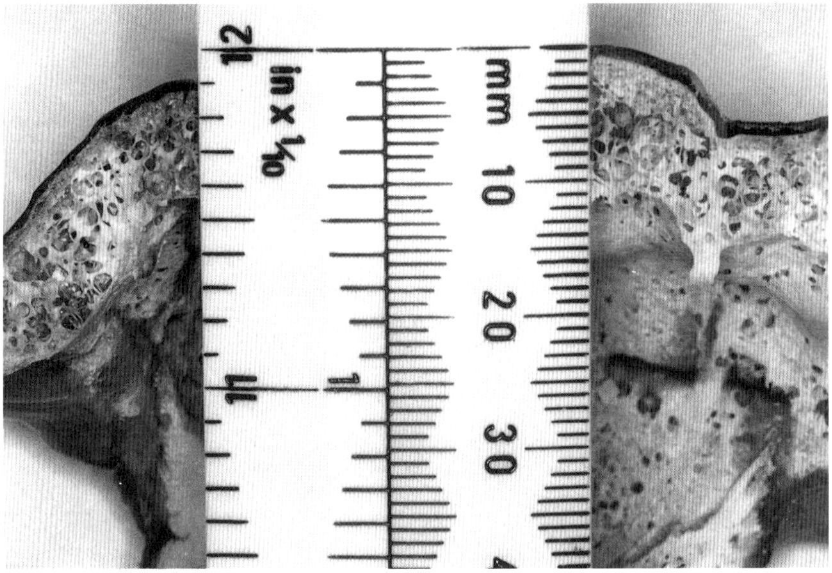


(a)

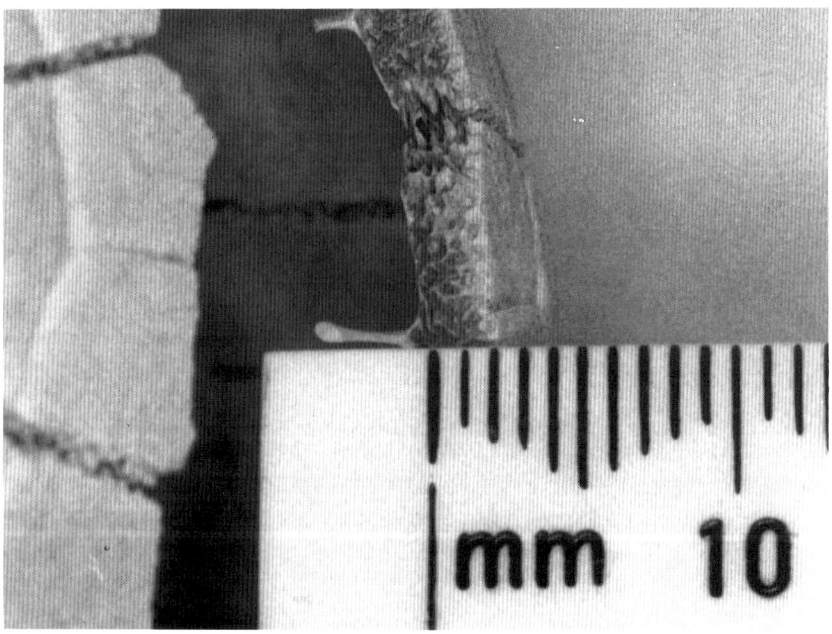


(b)

**Plate 7** The effects of high protein diets during periods of growth. The carapace thickness and texture of the two cross sections are notably different. (a) The carapace of a tortoise fed regularly with significant amounts of animal protein is five times thicker than (b) the equivalent animal fed on a herbivorous diet. The texture of the abnormal carapace is like that of an aerated chocolate bar! (Courtesy of A. Highfield.)

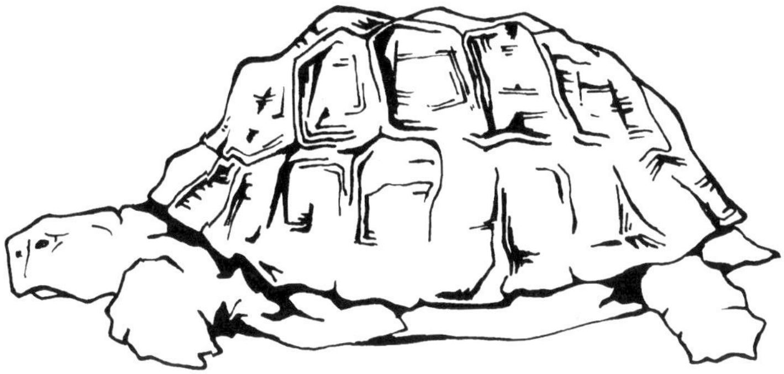

**Fig. 17** Moderate protein levels during times of growth results in even growth of the carapace.

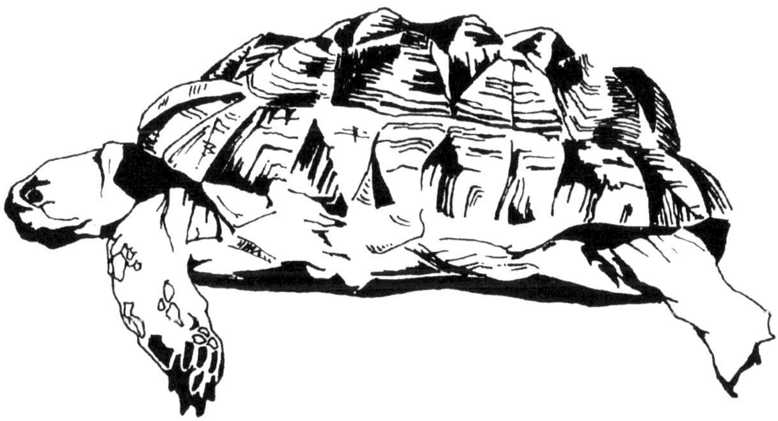

**Fig. 18** Excessive protein levels during times of growth results in overgrowth of horny tissue and pyramiding of the scutes.

# HELMINTH INFECTIONS

Nematodes are common parasites of Chelonia (Plate 8). Routine worming of tortoises is therefore recommended. Tortoises kept in colonies and those who endure poor hygiene are obviously more susceptible to this type of infection. Similarly reinfection post treatment will be more likely for these animals. Isolated animals once wormed, if kept hygienically, have a low likelihood of reinfection. High-risk animals would benefit from biannual worming, low-risk animals annual worming. Commonly found nematodes include:

- Ascarids – *Angusticaecum* sp.
- Oxyurids – *Tachygonetria* sp. and *Atractis dactyluris*.

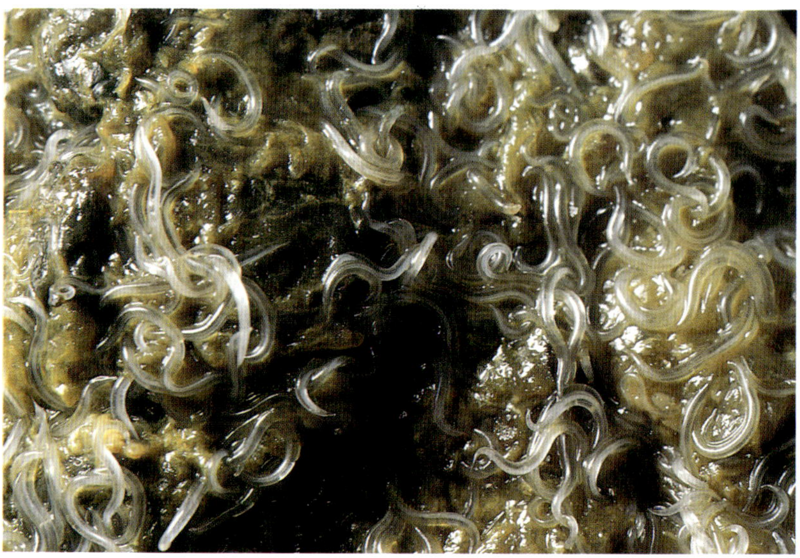

**Plate 8** Nematodes evacuated from newly imported pancake tortoise. (© A.C. Highfield.)

## SYMPTOMS

Affected animals are usually symptomless but sometimes animals with heavy worm burdens show anorexia, vomit worms and can lose condition. Secondary diarrhoea/enteritis or even impaction or obstruction may be observed.

## DIAGNOSIS

- Usually based upon observation of worms in faeces by the client.
- Faecal egg counts are worthwhile if helminths are suspected.
- Tortoises with a worm burden will obviously pass these after routine worming.

## TREATMENT

| Drug | Dose and frequency | Information on administration |
|---|---|---|
| **Oxfendazole** (e.g. Systemex: Mallinckrodt) | 65 mg/kg orally, as a single dose | Dosing is best achieved orally by passing a stomach tube and syringing in the treatment slowly (see section on 'Handling techniques'). As the dose can be quite large (3 ml/kg) it would appear to be sensible to give this volume gradually, perhaps even in smaller amounts spread over a short period of time. A single worming is usually all that is required. |
| **Fenbendazole** (e.g. Panacur: Hoechst) | 50–100 mg/kg orally, repeat in two weeks | Fenbendazole is also regularly used and is available in 5% and 10% solutions. This drug, like the above, has a wide safety margin but is not quite as effective as oxfendazole. Two doses 14 days apart are required, once again these are best given orally (see 'stomach tubing and oral dosing a tortoise' in the section on 'Handling techniques'). Both these wormings can be administered slowly by a client. Worm more frequently if worms or eggs continue to be observed. |

### Ivermectin

Though of great use in other species ivermectin has proved consistently fatal in Chelonia and is ***contraindicated*** (Teare & Bush 1983).

### Piperazine

Although recommended in some early publications on tortoises it is now considered ***toxic***. Products such as dog worming tablets or powders should be avoided, especially products purchased by the client from pet shops. Animals treated with moderate doses often survive but they may also still have their original worm burden.

## TAPEWORM INFECTIONS

These are not generally encountered in Mediterranean tortoises as they are herbivorous. Any intermediate host required would not be present. Infestations in recently imported omnivorous animals (should they be encountered) would probably respond to oxfendazole as previously described. Apparently a paper by Funk (1988) in the *Bulletin of Chicago Herpetological Society*, **23** (2), 30, suggests that Droncit: Bayer may be effective at 5–8 mg/kg i.m. without side effects but I have not seen this paper or used the drug myself (K. Fletcher, personal communication 1995).

# ECTOPARASITES

## TICKS

These are rarely encountered in the UK but, in view of the recent trends in importation of non-licensed species, it is possible for the veterinary surgeon to encounter ticks in recently imported animals (Plate 9). Petney & Knight (1988) document the use of a dilute Amitraz solution (e.g. Aludex: Hoechst) to successfully eliminate ticks during natural infection in a natural environment. A dose of 2 ml/litre was used and no adverse reactions were reported. Tick detachment was achieved.

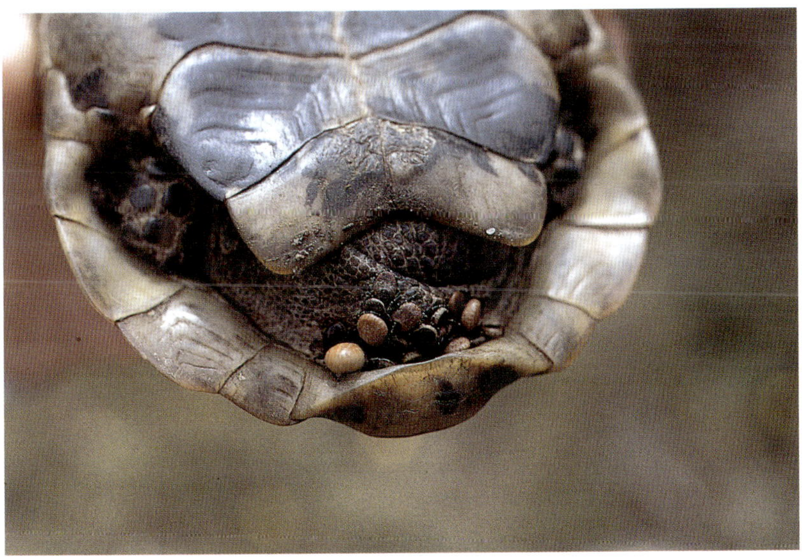

**Plate 9** Ticks (*Hyaloma* spp.) on a tortoise. In the wild frequently associated with grazing livestock. (© A.C. Highfield.)

## FLY STRIKE (MYIASIS)

Several authors have described treatment of affected animals (Gould & Georgi (1991); Frye (1991); Cooper & Jackson (1981), etc.) and this typically involves manual removal of larvae and thorough cleansing of the tissues with a disinfecting solution (e.g. povidone–iodine (Pevidine: C-Vet) or dilute hydrogen peroxide solution). It should be borne in mind that fly strike is usually a secondary problem and any predisposing cause such as cloacitis or trauma will require thorough investigation and treatment. Plate 10 shows fly strike on a Mediterranean tortoise.

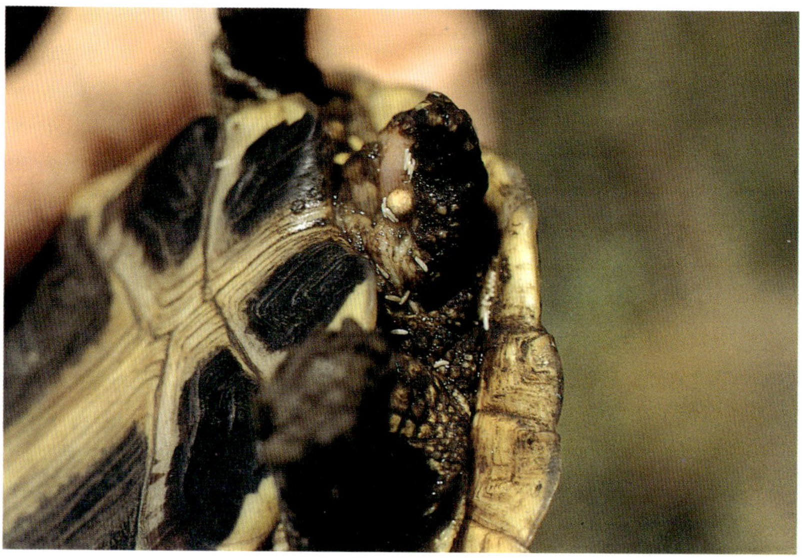

**Plate 10** Fly strike on the infected tail region of a Mediterranean tortoise (*Testudo hermanni*). (© A.C. Highfield.)

Ectoparasitides are not usually indicated if the underlying lesions are managed appropriately during their healing. Local application of antibiotics may be required, e.g. gentamicin ointment or cream. Systemic antibiotics may be appropriate if tissue infection has become extensive.

I have been informed that a visceral form of fly strike is occasionally seen in recently imported box tortoises. These are seen as swellings below the skin that burst to reveal emerging fly larvae. The larvae are described as being about the size of a grain of rice and treatment is usually manual removal/expression (K. Fletcher, personal communication 1995).

# BACTERIAL INFECTIONS

## CULTURE AND SENSITIVITY TESTING

- Many of the antibiotics suggested later are not routinely used in sensitivity testing. It may be worth advising a laboratory of suitable antibiotics for tortoises, particularly those immediately available within the practice. Suggestions can be found in the treatment boxes included with each condition.
- Without a sensitivity result one can always start treatment of an assumed bacterial infection with what appears to be the most promising antibiotic. This can be changed to a specific narrow spectrum antibiotic when the appropriate information is available.

## ISOLATION OF INFECTIONS

Many of the conditions discussed are highly infectious in nature. It is most important that such animals are isolated from all others and routine disinfection procedures are followed. Resistant or unusual infections contaminate sterile operating areas. Tortoise infections regularly fall into this category. Handwashing after handling these animals should be encouraged.

## TREATMENT BY CLIENTS/LAY PEOPLE

Many antibiotic injections are given every second day and the duration of antibiotic courses is often long, e.g. seven or more doses. If a veterinary surgeon has supervised a client injecting antibiotic solution correctly into their tortoise it may become possible for clients to be dispensed syringes, needles and antibiotics in order to inject into the patient themselves. The veterinary surgeon should arrange regular follow-up consultations to monitor progress. Few non-specialist vets have the time and patience to hospitalize a tortoise for long periods of time. The environmental conditions required are quite demanding if a suitable vivarium is not to hand.

I have also tried oral preparations of enrofloxacin (Baytril: Bayer) using a 1:5 dilution of a 2.5% solution in tortoises with very encouraging results, an oral antibiotic with low side effects would make treatment of chronic conditions far more practical. As enrofloxacin is quite alkali it is essential to dilute it before administration.

## STERILE GUT SYNDROME (SGS)

This is an unfortunate consequence of broad spectrum antibiotic therapy in a herbivorous animal dependent on favourable intestinal flora. Oxytetracycline given at or above 50 mg/kg is often implicated but it is possible with any antibiotic treatment, particularly if prolonged and broad spectrum. Apparently it seldom happens at lower doses such as 10 mg/kg (K. Fletcher, personal communication). Whilst antibiotics should be used sparingly, if the condition requires them, then they must be given despite the risk. Sterile gut syndrome is seen very infrequently, but it is serious when encountered.

### Symptoms

An intense diarrhoea with few bacteria upon faecal culture. Food is often passed undigested.

### Treatment

Specific treatment would logically consist of probiotics, although no literature appears available to endorse their efficacy.

**Possible probiotic sources include**

- Back-feeding faeces from a healthy tortoise of the same group (or faeces from the same tortoise, taken prior to treatment).
- Vetrumex (Willows Francis), Avipro, or similar.
- Live natural yoghurt as a small initial seeding dose of non-pathogenic organisms.

Page & Mautino (1990), using dose rates calculated during their earlier studies, have suggested that oral ketoconazole at a dose rate of 15–30 mg/kg daily will help prevent fungal superinfections during antiobitic therapy that alters gut flora. Similarly the use of culture and sensitivity to reveal the most appropriate and narrow spectrum antibiotic suitable, will help prevent the changes to commensal organisms when broad-spectrum therapy is administered.

Kaolin preparations such as Kaopectate: Upjohn may also be tried at 1 ml/kg twice daily.

## SALMONELLOSIS

This is not commonly encountered in herbivorous Chelonia, although there are various references to the disease being diagnosed in carnivorous and omnivorous species of turtles or terrapins that are kept in poor conditions. The serious risk of subsequent human infection makes animals known to have suffered this disease unsuitable as pets. This is important where children, the elderly, or immunosuppressed individuals are involved. Few carrier animals show symptoms of infection although diarrhoea and septicaemia are both possible. It is essential to maintain high levels of hand washing in clients dealing with these animals. This is also true of animals not suspected of having the disease.

Bolser (1988) discussed the epidemiology of salmonellosis in pet turtles, particularly *Pseudemys scripta elegans* (the common red-eared terrapin). Although the incidence of the disease is low in such reptiles, its importance as a serious zoonosis and the fact that the primary age group at risk is children, mean it must be considered a serious health hazard. Bolser stresses that it is not possible to identify an animal as being free of this disease and she advises that these animals should always be kept hygienically and preferably not by children. The disease risk is mainly associated with aquatic environments and carnivorous species. Mediterranean tortoises are unlikely to have this disease.

Animals treated for salmonella infections may well become carriers and should not be kept as pets if at all possible.

Zwart (1987) described a treatment for *Salmonella* spp. and *Campylobacter* spp. infections using a combination of ampicillin at 75 mg/tortoise and chloramphenicol at 250 mg/tortoise for ten days. Culture and sensitivity tests should be performed in order to find the most effective treatment available.

## RUNNY NOSE SYNDROME (RNS)

A rhinitis of, as yet, uncertain aetiology. Various contribution factors have been suggested by a variety of authors.

| **Possible contributing factors** |
|---|
| • *Mycoplasma* or *Chlamydia* infection<br>• Vitamin A deficiency<br>• Overcrowding, stress<br>• Inappropriate temperatures<br>• Inappropriate humidity<br>• Viral infection<br>• Mycosis<br>• Irritation from dust/spores |

Primary or secondary bacterial infections lead to a chronic, debilitating infection. Various bacteria have been isolated and these are usually Gram-negative (Holt *et al.* 1979; Lawrence & Needham 1985). Recent papers such as Vanrompay *et al.* (1994) indicate that *Chlamydia psittaci* may be involved.

| **Possible pathogenic bacteria** |
|---|
| • *Klebsiella* spp.<br>• *Pseudomonas* spp.<br>• *Citrobacter* spp.<br>• *Alikaligenes faecalis*<br>• *Staphylococcus aureus* |

*Testudo graeca*, the spur-thighed North African tortoise, may be predisposed to this condition (Jackson & Needham 1983, personal observation; The Tortoise Trust, personal communication). The pattern of spread of this disease amongst single species and mixed species colonies has been the subject of much investigation recently. The cause appears multifactorial because not all members of a colony of any type will contact the problem, immunity may have a role here. It is essential that great care is taken when groups of tortoises are mixed as this disease has caused significant problems when one colony is temporarily mixed with another (e.g. during tortoise sitting when an owner is on holiday). As carrier animals may exist, it seems sensible to try and maintain closed groups of similar origin animals in order to minimize this and other diseases, such as necrotic stomatitis, that may be related.

### Treatment

- Isolate affected animals.
- Correct any nutritional or environmental problems (especially humidity).

- Check for nasal foreign body.
- Take a swab for culture and sensitivity (? include a chlamydial transport medium).
- Apply antibiotics as appropriate.
- Continued supportive treatment such as good nutrition, hydration, and suitable environmental management.

> A useful method of antibiotic application involves breaking off a 21G needle at its hub. This new needle can be used to apply two drops of undiluted oxytetracycline injection (e.g. Terramycin Q50: Pfizer Ltd) directly into the nasal chambers, as it fits the external nares perfectly. Treatment is given daily and often an improvement is seen within a week. Other antibiotic drops used include neomycin and tobramycin. Lawrence & Needham (1985) discussed a good response to tylosin and suggested *Chlamydia* or *Mycoplasma* infection may be present. Enrofloxacin (Baytril: Bayer) is currently being tried with good results at a dose rate of 2.5–5.0 mg/kg i.m. daily (Dorrestein 1992) supporting this theory.

### Prognosis

Some infections in individuals are persistent despite treatment. This may be due to non-healing ulcers in the nasal chambers or due to environmental problems, e.g. unsuitable humidity. It is wise to avoid the use of steroids in any drops applied as this might delay the healing of such lesions. It is possible that carrier animals may exist.

## NECROTIC STOMATITIS

This is well described by many authors such as Holt *et al.* (1979). It is a necrotic infection of the buccal cavity usually affecting the mucous membrane of the labia, gingiva and glossa with associated diphtheric membrane formation (Plate 11). The disease is common in recently hibernated tortoises as hibernation allows optimal conditions for the disease to progress. It is a major complication of post-hibernation anorexia (PHA).

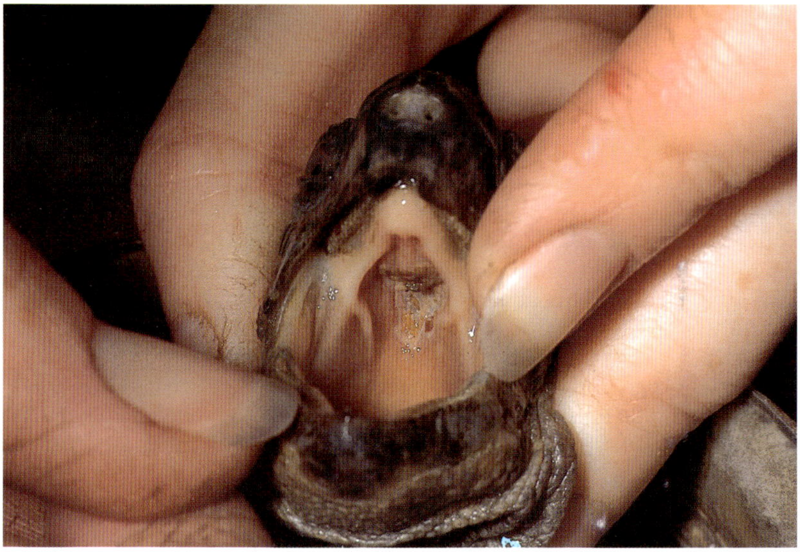

**Plate 11** An unusual presentation of 'mouth rot' or necrotic stomatitis in the upper palate of *Testudo graeca*. Nasal lesions are also present at the external nares. (© A.C. Highfield.)

## Aetiology

**Possible contributing factors**

- *Pseudomonas* spp.
- *Aeromonas* spp.
- Possible *Mycoplasma/Chlamydia* involvement.
- Further bacteria (e.g. *Beta haemolytic E. coli*).
- Possible primary viral infection.
- Chronic vitamin A deficiency affecting epithelial integrity.
- Debility/hibernation of debilitated animals.
- Hibernation of animals which have recently eaten.

There is a shortage of conclusive information defining the true aetiology of this condition. Cooper *et al.* (1988) record the presence of herpes-like particles in post-mortem cases in *T. graeca* and include information by other authors linking herpes virus with glossitis, septicaemia and meningoencephalitis. Chlamydial or similar agents may also be involved.

## Symptoms

- Presenting symptoms include anorexia (presumably due to mouth pain), recurrent mouth opening and facial swelling. The condition has been seen to occur in combination with runny nose syndrome and deaths in the early post-hibernation period. The most obvious finding is a white necrotic diphtheric membrane formation, particularly on the tongue. Early cases may have haemorrhagic foci or just appear erythematous. A swab rubbed gently around the mouth and over the tongue often results in a sloughing of gingival and glossal epithelium. Severe cases can involved an osteomyelitis of the jaw and carry a very guarded prognosis.

- It should be noted that animals sharing the same feeding areas and those in poor hygiene are at great risk from affected companions. All affected animals require strict isolation. The history of an outbreak commonly includes exposure of animals to tortoises from different backgrounds, such as during holiday 'tortoise sitting' or the acquisition of new animals. The possibility that carriers may exist should be considered.

## Diagnosis

Usually based on history and clinical examination, although swabs from affected and in-contact animals can be of great use. The lesions are pathognomonic.

## Treatment

All affected animals should be isolated from other healthy stock. Treatment depends on the severity of the condition.

| A treatment plan for necrotic stomatitis | Advice on procedure |
|---|---|
| • Isolate affected animals correct any environmental or nutritional problems. | |
| • Take a swab for culture and sensitivity. | |
| • Debride mouth (possibly with anaesthesia as this is painful). | Use a cotton swab. |
| • Local disinfection with povidone-iodine solution (e.g. Pevidine: C-Vet). | Use a cotton swab. |
| • Continue daily cleaning/oral hygiene. | |

| A treatment plan for necrotic stomatitis | Advice on procedure |
|---|---|
| • Undertake supportive treatment such as stomach tubing and rehydration. Severe cases may require a pharyngostomy or naso gastric tube. | ***Stomach tubes should be passed only once the mouth has been packed with a suitable antibacterial preparation, otherwise any infection will be spread down the oesophagus.*** |
| • Severe cases may require antibiotic therapy. | Framomycin: C-Vet locally in paste form is very effective. It can also be supplemented systemically at <10 mg/kg. Care should be taken as it is a nephrotoxic aminoglycoside. (See the section on 'Drugs and Dosages'.) Systemic antibiotics are not always indicated, unless it is feared that the infection is advancing to a septicaemia. Enrofloxacin (Baytril: Bayer) has proved of great use in severe cases. |
| • Acyclovir ointment 5% (Zovirax: Wellcome) has been used with good results in cases assumed to have a primary viral aetiology (Cooper *et al.* 1988). | |

### Prognosis

This is hard to predict. It is good if treated early but the condition can become chronic. Results personally observed have varied from rapid death to full recovery.

## PNEUMONIA

The anatomy of the chelonian respiratory system is somewhat different to that of mammals. The lungs are situated dorsally just below the carapace (Fig. 19) and do not possess true pleural membranes. They have the texture and appearance of sponge. A horizontal membrane is present and its movements influence lung ventilation. Inflation is aided by limb movement.

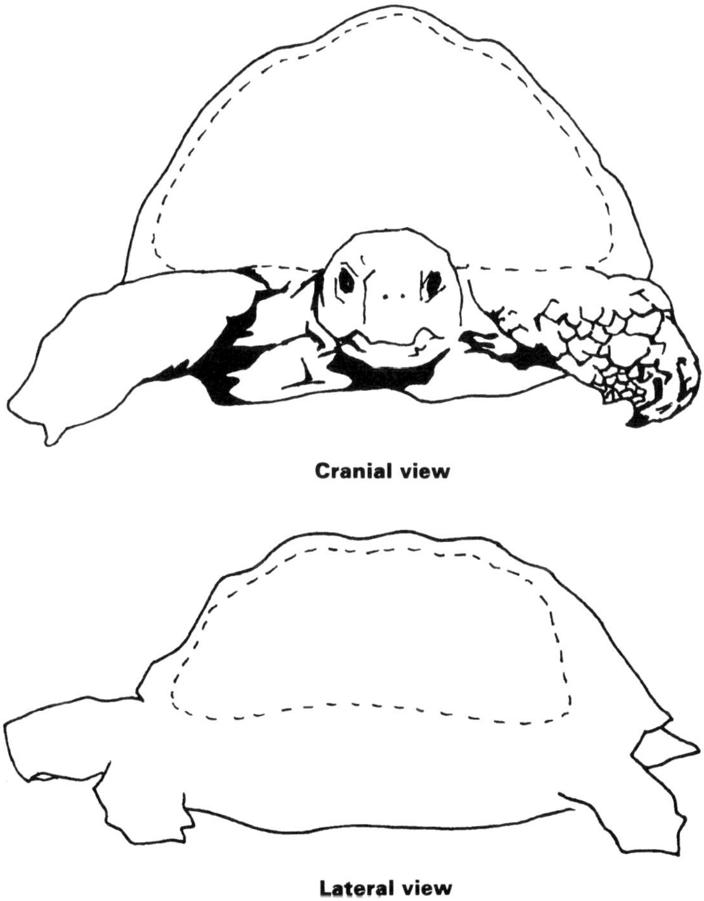


**Fig. 19** A lateral and cranial view showing the area occupied by the lung fields.

## ACUTE PNEUMONIA

This disease can progress rapidly to death within just a few hours. If this initial period is survived it may develop into the chronic form. It is quite likely that the acute form of the disease has a primary causal agent, e.g. *Chlamydia psittaci* (Vanrompay *et al.* 1994) or possibly a virus, with secondary bacterial involvement.

### Symptoms

| Signs of acute pneumonia |
|---|
| • Gaping of the mouth/neck-stretching<br>• Excessive nasal/oral discharge<br>• Cyanosis/weakness<br>• Hyperactivity (because of respiratory distress)<br>• Concurrent disease (e.g. necrotic stomatitis, hepatitis/jaundice) |

### Treatment

| A treatment plan for acute pneumonia | Examples of suitable antibiotics |
|---|---|
| • Isolate affected animals.<br>• Deliver injectable antibiotics (i.v. if possible).<br>• Maintaining a high body temperature may increase antibiotic activity and stimulate immunity (30°C).<br>• Affected animals should be rehydrated using a stomach tube and rehydration preparation (e.g. Lectade: SmithKline Beecham). | • Enrofloxacin (e.g. Baytril: Bayer 2.5–5.0 mg/kg i.m. or i.v.)<br>• Ampicillin (e.g. Penbritin: SmithKline Beecham 50 mg/kg i.m.)<br>• Oxytetracycline (various, 50 mg/kg i.m.)<br>• Tylosin (e.g. Tylan 50: Elanco 25–50 mg/kg i.m.)<br>*Mycoplasma/Chlamydia* infections would be controlled with enrofloxacin or tylosin should these agents be implicated in the aetiology. |

### Prognosis

This must be guarded, but affected animals may recover if treated quickly. The aetiology needs more thorough investigation and the causal agents and species affected may prove to affect the progress of the disease.

## CHRONIC PNEUMONIA

Where chronic pneumonia exists the radiographic and surgical drilling techniques described in later sections may be the only effective method of dealing with the problem. The prognosis in such animals is not normally very good.

Lesions can often be located using a combination of lateral and dorso-ventral radiographs and in extreme cases this information can be used to drill through the carapace, swab lung lesions and place the appropriate antibiotic directly onto the infection.

A drill hole requires plugging between treatments, possibly with sterile Blu-tac®, in order to allow respiratory function to be continued. Analgesia must be considered when drilling the access hole and care must be taken to prevent foreign material entering through this hole.

### Symptoms

| Signs of chronic pneumonia |
|---|
| • Persistent, low level mucous discharge from mouth<br>• Cyanosis (mauve mucous membranes)<br>• Generalized weakness<br>• Sometimes rocking and recurrent mouth opening are seen<br>• Concurrent disease |

### Treatment

| A treatment plan for chronic pneumonia |
|---|
| • An oropharyngeal swab for culture and sensitivity or if possible a swab taken from lung tissue via a drill hole.<br>• Enrofloxacin, aminoglycoside or other antibiotics according to sensitivity (e.g. Baytril: Bayer at 5 mg/kg daily or gentamicin or Framomycin: C-Vet at 10 mg/kg every 40 hours for about seven doses: see 'Therapeutics').<br>• Shell drilling and introduction of local antibiotics through the resulting hole if a poor response to above.<br>• Appropriate supportive therapy (e.g. fluid administration). |

### Prognosis

Many cases are reported to respond to antibiotic injections but some cases respond poorly and die, or show recurrence.

## OCULAR INFECTIONS AND RELATED CONDITIONS

Conjunctivitis and blepharatis occur frequently. Hypovitaminosis A predisposes to the condition and occasionally blepharitis can be the result of an ascending infection from an ear abscess, oropharyngeal infection, or even foreign body irritation. Infectious bacterial superficial keratitis appears as a small white blob on the corneal surface and responds well to appropriate antibiosis.

## Treatment

This consists of correction of nutrition if required, appropriate treatment of concurrent disease and topical antibiotics. These antibiotics include:

- Cloxacillin (e.g. Orbenin: SmithKline Beecham)
- Neomycin (e.g. Neobiotic: Upjohn)
- Gentamicin (e.g. Genticin: Roche)
- Chloramphenicol (e.g. Chloromycetin: Parke Davis)
- Tobramycin (e.g. Tobralex: Alcon)

The duration of the course depends upon the severity of the condition; it should extend beyond visual clinical recovery. Most ointments can be given four to six times daily.

| | |
|---|---|
| **Ocular foreign bodies** | These tend to be introduced behind the nictitating membrane by the forelegs during feeding. They should be removed with anaesthesia if necessary, and subsequent antibiotic therapy given if required. |
| **Cataracts and damage to nervous tissue** | These are also common particularly in frost damaged animals but treatment is probably beyond the scope of the general practitioner. Clinics with eye specialists and suitable equipment may wish to try lens extraction if lens opacity is present, but this has yet to be documented as a viable procedure in this species. Some frost damaged animals will regain sight in time if nursed and force fed as required. This may take as long as two years. Some animals will also be brain damaged from the same temperature insult. |

## Prognosis

Usually quite good. Chronic untreated eye infections often rupture and abscessate requiring surgical enucleation.

## CLOACITIS

An inflamed or ulcerated cloacal opening with resultant discharge. May be secondary to a cloacal calculus, egg retention or a parasite burden.

**A treatment plan for cloacitis**

- Check for calculus or egg retention and provide appropriate treatment.
- Screen for protozoa/helminthiasis.
- Flush the cloaca with povidone-iodine (Pevidine: C-Vet).
- Possibly flush the cloaca with antibiotic paste (e.g. Framomycin: C-Vet).

### Prognosis

Good provided any underlying cause is removed.

## ULCERATIVE SHELL DISEASE (USD)

Plates 12–14 show examples of ulcerative shell disease. There are two forms of this disease: wet USD and dry USD.

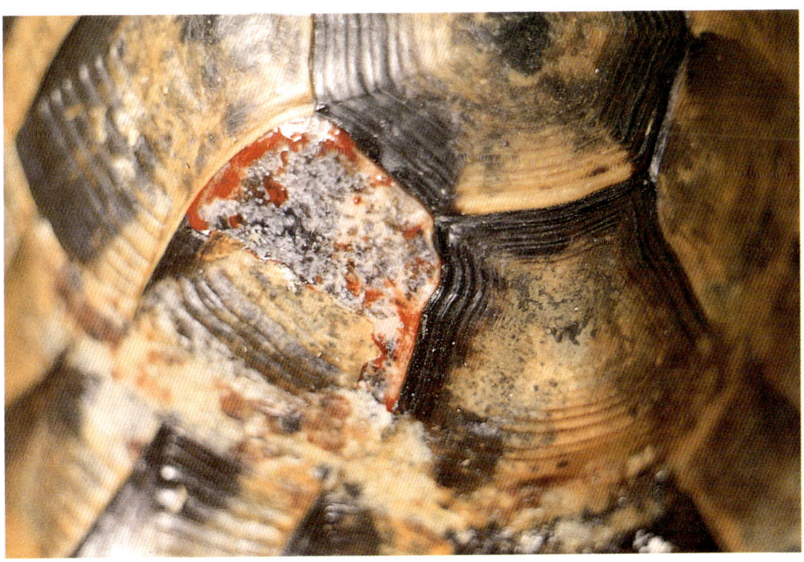

**Plate 12** 'Wet' or bacterial, shell rot. (© A.C. Highfield.)

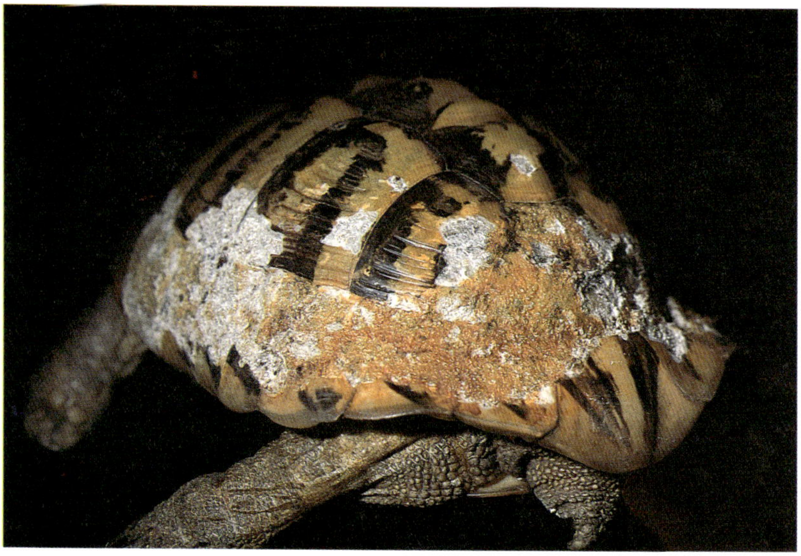

**Plate 13** 'Dry' variety of necrotic dermatitis (shell rot or USD). (© A.C. Highfield.)

| | Wet USD | Dry USD |
|---|---|---|
| **Aetiology** | Bacterial in origin:<br>• *Pseudomonas* spp.<br>• *Citrobacter* spp.<br>• *Klebsiella* spp. | Fungal in origin:<br>• Mixed bacterial/ fungal infections are also possible.<br>• It can become a chronic problem. |
| **Symptoms** | • A foul smelling haemorrhagic discharge from between the scutes.<br>• The infection tends to spread laterally under the scutes causing their attachments to the underlying bone to be weakened.<br>• Such scutes are easily lifted off.<br>• Wet USD is a potential emergency. It often predisposes to a peracute and fatal septicaemia following the initial infection. It may also spread to involve the skin.<br>• This is occasionally referred to as SCUD, especially in soft-shelled turtles. This disease may also have viral or mycoplasma aetiology. | • It may present as lifting and flaking of the scutes. |

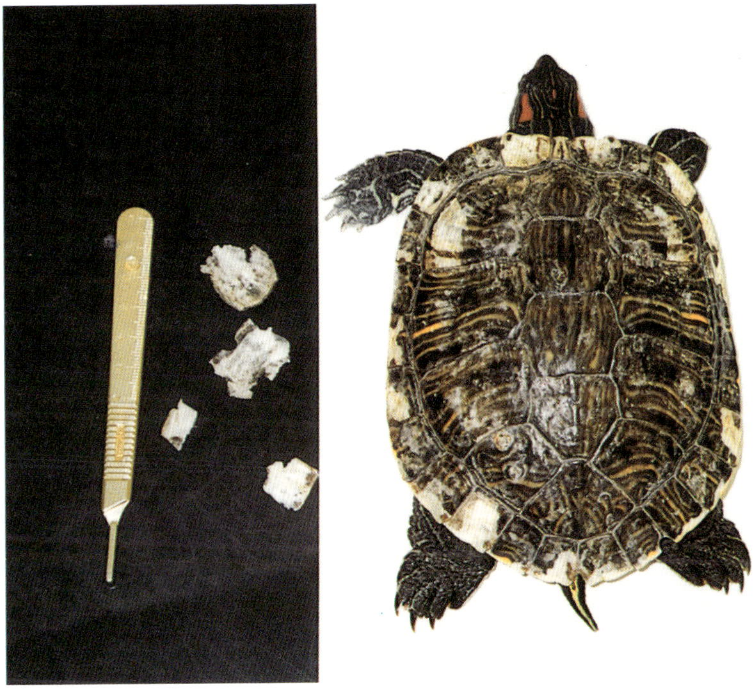

(a)

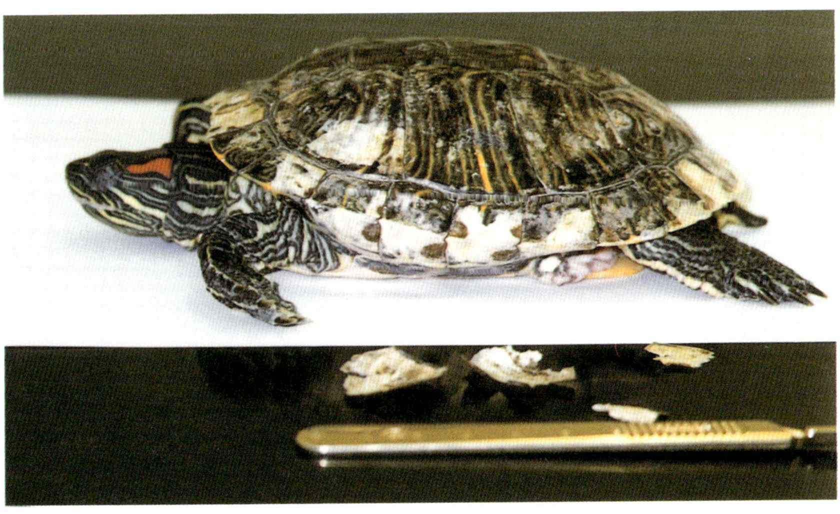

(b)

**Plate 14** Ulcerative shell disease in a four-year-old red-eared slider. (a) Dorsal view and (b) lateral view. This animal was euthanased after five months of treatment.

**A treatment plan for USD**

- Remove any affected shell material to allow exposure to air. This infection mainly thrives at low oxygen concentrations.
- In terrapins reducing contact with water is beneficial.
- Swab the affected area for aerobic and anaerobic infections. Undertake culture and sensitivity testing.
- Debride the area with a povidone-iodine solution (e.g. Pevidine: C-Vet) and apply this in concentrated form daily. Oxygenating agents such as dilute hydrogen peroxide may be of use in the first stages of treatment (later they may delay healing).
- After extensive debridement, the affected area can be treated with a topical antibiotic according to the sensitivity result. The aminoglycosides are very effective and good results have been achieved with:
    - Framomycin paste (C-Vet)
    - Gentamicin ointment/cream (e.g. Genticin: Roche)
    - Silver sulphadiazine (e.g. Flamazine: Smith & Nephew).
- Parenteral use of antibiotics according to sensitivity (e.g. enrofloxacin (Baytril: Bayer)).
- Exposure of affected areas to oxygen/air is often the most fruitful line of treatment. This may well mean that extensive removal of scutes is required. Such animals must not be hibernated until this damage is suitably repaired.

## SEPTICAEMIA

This is not uncommon (Plate 15). Two common bacteria involved are *Pseudomonas* spp. and *Aeromonas* spp., but others are also possible.

Septicaemia is often the result of a bacterial infection such as pneumonia, ulcerative shell disease or abscess reaching the blood stream. Viral and chlamydial immunosuppression have been suggested as factors predisposing to septicaemia but this still requires appropriate confirmation.

**Symptoms of septicaemia may include**

- Vomiting
- Lethargy
- Erythematous flush to plastron and carapace
- Secondary jaundice (yellowed mucous membranes)
- Polydipsia
- Petechial haemorrhages of the mucus membranes (esp. mouth)

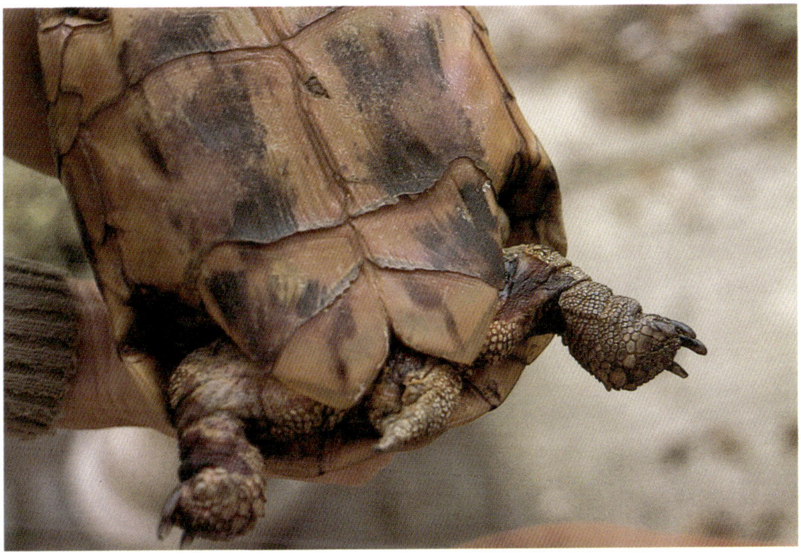

**Plate 15** The plastron of a tortoise affected by acute septicaemia. (© A.C. Highfield.)

**A treatment plan for septicaemia**

- Deliver injectable antibiotics as quickly as possible, e.g.

| | |
|---|---|
| Enrofloxacin | 2.5–5 mg/kg i.m. daily |
| Framycetin | 10 mg/kg i.m. 48–72 hourly |
| Gentamicin | 10 mg/kg i.m. 48–72 hourly |
| Oxytetracycline | 50 mg/kg i.m. daily |
| Ampicillin | 50 mg/kg i.m. daily |

- Appropriate fluid therapy should be undertaken.
- Animals should be maintained at a temperature appropriate to the antibiotic.

### Prognosis

Guarded.

## PERITONITIS

This condition often presents in a similar manner as septicaemia.

| **Common causes of peritonitis** |
| --- |
| • Egg retention and secondary rupture of an oviduct |
| • Perforation of intestine by worm burden |
| • Renal, cloacal, or other calculi |

The peritonitis requires an appropriate antibiotic but the underlying cause should also be treated (see the sections on 'Helminth infections', 'Surgical techniques and shell repairs' etc.).

In view of the seriousness of the causes of peritonitis a very poor prognosis is usually given.

## SEPTIC ARTHRITIS

This may in fact be several conditions collected under one title. Some septic arthritis cases appear sterile on culture and it is possible that these stem from either a fungal problem or an 'articular gout' as a result of excessive dietary protein intake, or a period of impaired renal function.

### Symptoms

- Swelling of one or more legs.
- Stiffening of the joints.
- Radiography is useful to determine the extent of the disease.

### Treatment

| Medical management | Surgical amputation of the affected limb |
| --- | --- |
| • If in the early stages systemic antibiotics may prove effective.<br>• The following have been suggested by some authors:<br>○ Enrofloxacin (Baytril: Bayer) 2.5–5 mg/kg i.m. daily<br>○ Gentamicin (e.g. Genticin: Roche) <10 mg/kg 48–72 hours at 24°C<br>○ Framycetin (e.g. Framomycin 5%: C-Vet) <10 mg/kg 48–72 hours at 24°C<br>○ Oxytetracycline (e.g. Terramycin Q50: Pfizer Ltd) 50 mg/kg i.m.<br>• The duration of treatment will depend on the severity of the problem.<br>• It must be remembered that reptiles have slow rates of healing. | • High amputations are required as stumps become traumatized and wound breakdown will occur.<br>• Forelegs tend to be easier than hind legs (see advice on 'Surgical techniques and shell repair').<br>• This is the treatment of choice if radiography indicates that bone is involved.<br>• It is currently in vogue to use Lego® wheels affixed to the plastron adjacent to the site of amputation with epoxy adhesive as a form of prosthesis. This is not often required.<br>• Careful follow-up is vital. |

### Prognosis

Guarded, but depends on the extent of the problem and possible surgical complications. Obviously post-operative checks should be extensive.

## EAR ABSCESSES

This is often seen as swelling of the tympanic scale, an obvious anatomical feature. Usually, though *not always* unilateral. The abscess may discharge through the eustachian tube into the back of the throat, result in a surrounding cellulitis, or become hard and inspissated. I have even seen this type of infection in very young tortoises of 60 g or less. Oro-faecal contamination has been implicated as a possible cause.

## Symptoms

These include anorexia, dysphagia, blepharitis, rubbing of the face and a distorted head shape (Fig. 20).

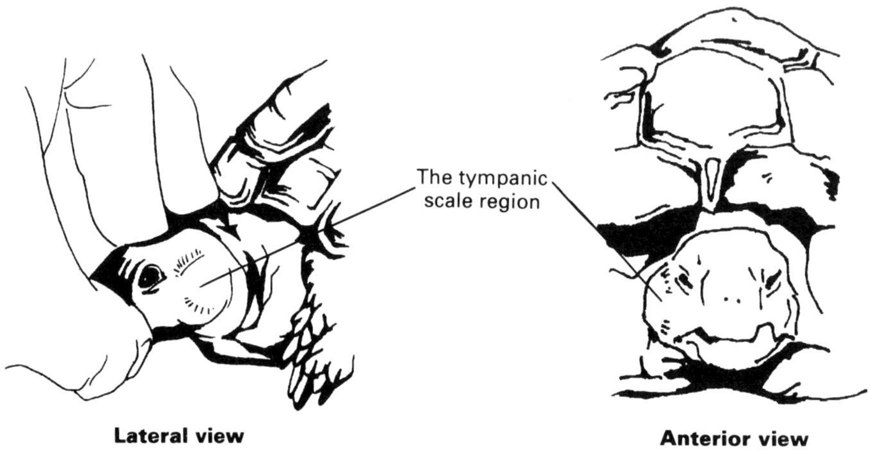


**Fig. 20** Ear abscesses. Ear abscesses may result in swelling of this region or inflammation that often progresses towards (and may include) the eye.

**A treatment plan for an aural abscess**

- Medical treatment with antibiotics on their own is not often successful as, whilst it may appear effective in the short term, a reservoir of infection tends to remain resulting in recurrence. There is a constant threat that the abscess will become active once more and disseminate. An inspissated abscess may also produce chronic pain or interfere with jaw opening.
- Curative treatment is usually surgical. The abscess is curetted, swabbed, and flushed and then packed with suitable antibiotic (anaesthesia is required). It is suggested that the abscess wall must also be surgically removed.
- Some authors advise suturing the tympanic scale post-operatively but I have found drainage and exposure to be of greater use. Recurrence appears to be common in sutured cases whereas in those cases which have been allowed to drain naturally and subjected to careful post-operative cleaning and monitoring, recurrent problems are much less frequent. Always check the pharynx for eustachian tube involvement.
- Postoperative antibiosis locally, e.g.:
  - Fucidin (Fucithalmic: Leo)
  - Framomycin paste (C-Vet), gentamicin (Genticin: Roche)
  - According to sensitivity.

- Systemic antibiotics according to sensitivity if infection does not respond to local treatment (e.g. enrofloxacin (Baytril: Bayer), etc.).
- Continued post-operative flushing, curettage and observation as required.
- Cryosurgery has been used with varying success by the author to treat resistant infections where no suitable antibiotic, following extensive sensitivity testing, was available.

## SUBCUTICULAR ABSCESSES

These are treated in much the same way as above but it is sometimes possible to excise these under local anaesthesia. Inspissated abscesses may shell out during palpation. If the infection is active, then complete surgical excision under general or local anaesthesia should be undertaken. Again the lesion may be sutured if removed in entirety.

| Bacteria isolated include | Sites of recorded abscesses include |
|---|---|
| • *Pseudomonas* spp. | • Ears |
| • *Aeromonas* spp. | • Legs (post-injection site abscesses are common) |
| • *Citrobacter* spp. | • Nasal passages |
| • *Proteus* spp. | • Jaw and associated tissues |
| • *Serratia* spp. | • Internal abscess |
| • *Enterobacter* spp. | • Tail, etc. |
| • *Klebsiella* spp. | |

Post-operative care and antibiotics as described above are essential.

### Prognosis

This is usually favourable but recovery can be prolonged and recurrence is possible.

# FUNGAL INFECTIONS

## EXTERNAL INFECTIONS

Dry ulcerative shell disease (USD) often has a fungal component to it. Symptoms tend to involve a lifting off, and perhaps crumbling, of scutes (see Plate 13).

## TREATMENT

- Debride and expose damaged shell.
- Swab if a bacterial component is suspected.
- Disinfect with povidone-iodine solution (Pevidine: C-Vet).
- Dressing with malachite green at 2 mg/litre and/or oxidizing agents such as hydrogen peroxide have been suggested.

If fungal or yeast infections are indicated by way of examination of discharges and swabs from skin or cloacal lesions, then preparations containing antifungal agents may be applied once or twice daily. Examples include:

- Panolog (containing nystatin): Ciba Animal Health
- Daktarin (containing miconizole): Janssen
- Timodine (containing nystatin): Reckitt and Coleman.

Preparations known to contain steroids should perhaps be avoided if immunosuppression is considered to play a role (unfortunately some of the above fall into this category). Povidone-iodine preparations, dilute hydrogen peroxide or ketoconazole-impregnated gauze dressings may be of use here.

## INTERNAL INFECTIONS

If internal mycosis is suspected, as in a chronic pneumonia, or chronic arthritis, cellulitis or dermatitis, then ketoconazole has been advised at a dose of 15–30 mg/kg orally per day by Page & Mautino (1990) with good success rates and minimal side effects.

## MYCOTIC ENTERITIS

This has been described by Zwart & Buitelaar (1980) who treated the condition effectively using nystatin (Panalog: Ciba Animal Health) at a dose of 0.2–0.3 ml daily orally. *Candida* spp. superinfections are not uncommon as a result of previous antibiotic therapy producing an unfavourable bacterial flora. Recent reports have suggested that the immunosuppressive effects of as yet unidentified viruses may also allow an animal to become overwhelmed by a superinfection of normal organisms. Until this subject has been thoroughly investigated it would be wise to consider isolating such animals from any others. The treatment suggested by Page & Mautino (1990) and Page *et al.* (1988), using oral ketoconazole, will probably be effective here. It has also been suggested that animals undergoing intensive antibiotic therapy be treated with ketoconazole in order to prevent an opportunist fungal superinfection from developing although I am not sure how necessary this really is.

# *MYCOPLASMA/CHLAMYDIA* DISEASES

Little published information is currently available on this subject, although a recent paper in the UK by Vanrompay *et al.* (1994) documents the isolation of *Chlamydia* in sick tortoises with mucopurulent bronchopneumonia. Hill (1985) isolated *Mycoplasma testudinis* from the cloaca of a spur-thighed tortoise. Several recent papers involving Elliot Jacobson also indicate the likelihood of serious *Mycoplasma/ Chlamydia* diseases in Chelonia.

It is certainly possible that commonly encountered diseases such as runny nose syndrome and necrotic stomatitis have a multifactorial aetiology involving these agents, possibly even as cofactors. Similarly there is anecdotal evidence to suggest that pneumonias and acute fatal epidemics also involve these agents. Antimicrobial agents such as tylosin and enrofloxacin (Baytril: Bayer) seem to have been used with encouraging results, supporting this hypothesis. This area of reptile medicine requires further research. Isolation of *Chlamydia* is not often attempted in sick tortoises due to complexity and expense.

Much of the information given for viral diseases with respect to isolation and spread of infections is also valid for *Mycoplasma/Chlamydia* type diseases, should they prove to exist.

# VIRAL INFECTIONS

It is possible that diseases such as runny nose syndrome, necrotic stomatitis, and some forms of pneumonia and hepatitis may have a viral agent underlying their primary pathology (Frye *et al.* (1977); Jackson & Needham (1983); Heldstab & Besetti (1982); Cooper *et al.* (1988); Lange *et al.* (1989); Oettle *et al.* (1990); Beynon *et al.* (1992); Jacobson (1994b)).

A herpes-type virus or particles with this appearance have been found in many cases so far investigated. Other viruses such as paramyxoviruses and sendiviruses have been proposed but conclusive reports are not yet available. Most isolations are reported for one or two cases only, due to lack of clinical material and the expense of virus identification.

Epidemiological studies of large scale epidemics in tortoise colonies in this and other countries also point to the likelihood of perhaps more serious viral/*Mycoplasma*/*Chlamydia* diseases in the tortoise.

Until specific details are understood, it seems only sensible to advise that tortoise colonies be kept closed as much as possible. New animals should be isolated for several months before they are introduced to a main group. It would be wise to mix these animals with a small number of 'sentinel' tortoises before they contact any of the larger group.

Captive-bred animals should be released into natural habitats with great caution especially if they have mixed with different species from different locations during their lives. It is wise to take precautions to prevent the introduction of infections into natural wild populations. Symptomless carriers may exist and all such introductions should be undertaken only after extensive investigation and must be monitored carefully thereafter. Large-scale fatal epidemic disease outbreaks among Gopher tortoises in the US (*Xerobates* sp.) have followed releases of ex-captive animals. This underlines the need for extreme care when allowing contact between wild and ex-captive animals.

There is currently much heated debate concerning the possibility of fatal viral epidemics in tortoise colonies. Fatal epidemics of unknown aetiology certainly do occur and are most alarming to the attending veterinary surgeon. However, it is not clear whether these have a viral aetiology or not. I have personally observed several epidemics where two populations of animals have been mixed whilst one owner was away on holiday. Death or serious illness occurred in about 50% of the animals. The duration of illness in animals which died was around 24–48 hours and the pathology included hepatitis, pneumonia and stomatitis at post-mortem examination (virus isolation was not available).

Similar reports are available:

- Oettle *et al.* (1990) who demonstrated both herpes virus-like inclusions and paramyxovirus-like inclusions in an episode of 31 deaths over six months in a well-managed tortoise colony. Epidemiological studies also implicated a virus-like infection.
- Lange *et al.* (1989) describe evidence of a herpes virus they implicate as the possible cause of 50% mortality in a group of 130 Hermann's tortoises and four-toed tortoises during a three-month disease epidemic in 1987. The post-mortem findings included lesions of the upper digestive tract, liver and lower digestive tract. Virus particles were only isolated from three animals and it was not possible to demonstrate pathogenicity in turtle embryonic tissue culture.
- Frye *et al.* (1977) described a fatal herpes virus-like infection in two Pacific pond turtles where virus particles were located in spleen, liver and kidney.
- Rebell *et al.* (1975) describe a herpes virus-type agent affecting young Green Sea turtle hatchlings and implicated it as being the cause of grey patch disease. The disease was transmitted by a bacteria-free preparation of virus particles.
- Haines & Kleese (1977) further investigated herpes virus grey patch disease and demonstrated how external stress factors, such as water temperature, affected mortality rates.
- Jacobson (1994) reviews much of the literature available on tortoise mortality and infectious diseases and documents a paper of his own that identifies herpes virus-like agents in Argentine tortoises during an episode where 1200 of 2200 recently imported tortoises died. He also discusses a large amount of literature that describes probable herpes virus, iridovirus, poxvirus and togavirus infections of tortoises.

Many of the instances cited do not prove the infectious agent to be conclusively viral. It is possible that infectious *Chlamydia/Mycoplasma* or other type diseases exist, perhaps even simultaneously with virus infections as cofactors.

Captive breeding of Chelonia of all types within large colonies or populations should be undertaken cautiously as it is possible that we could unknowingly encourage these agents.

Conservation projects such as those for the green, leatherback and other turtles and tortoises where headstarting of hatchlings is followed by release into contact with wild populations, provide a potential disease transmission route. This must be observed closely in order to prevent any possible introduction of disease into an endangered population that may have no prior natural immunity. Plate 16 shows viral disease in a hatchling loggerhead turtle.

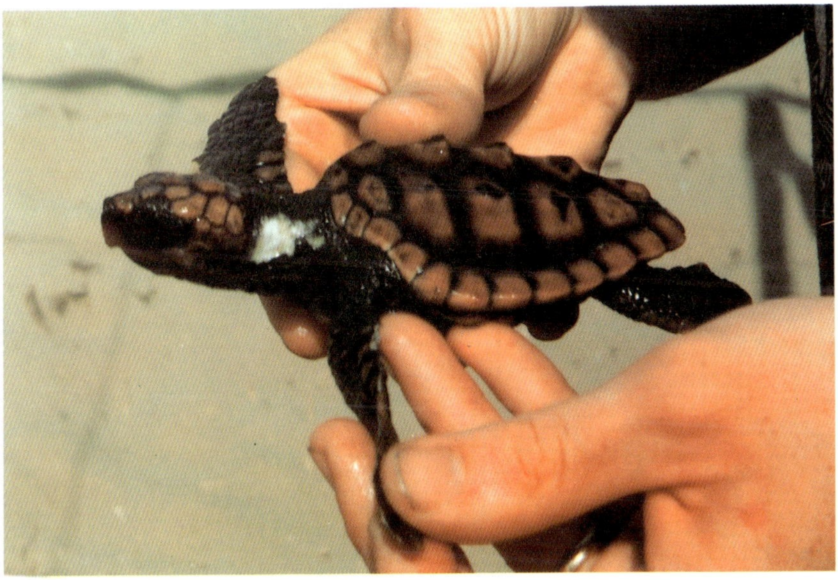

**Plate 16** Viral disease in a hatchling loggerhead turtle (*Caretta caretta*). Grey patch disease is now thought to be due to a herpes virus. The disease is prevalent in poor conditions of husbandry with poor water quality and overcrowding. In the outbreaks I have observed both morbidity and mortality rates were high and both green and loggerhead hatchlings were affected. Disease symptoms included grey sloughing skin lesions especially around the eyes, pharyngeal lesions, anorexia, wasting, jaundice and death. It is worrying that conservation breeding and reintroduction programmes may be releasing infected or carrier animals into the wild and exposing the already fragile and endangered wild populations of turtles to fatal diseases.

Cooper *et al.* (1991) tried to calm concern on this subject but still advised caution be taken when mixing groups of tortoises. They claim these epidemics have possibly always occurred and are not a new phenomenon, but do not consider the possibility that man may be encouraging them. They point out that viral immunosuppression in the tortoise has not yet been demonstrated. Investigations to understand this area of Chelonian medicine must continue.

Cooper *et al.* (1988) commented that some animals with necrotic stomatitis responded well to antiviral therapy Acyclovir 5% ointment (Zovirax: Wellcome) and a herpes or adenovirus infection was implicated. Interestingly isolations were all from *T. graeca* spp.

# PROTOZOAN AND COCCIDIAL INFECTIONS

## *HEXAMITA* INFECTION

A flagellate parasite of the urinary system that may lead to acute or chronic renal failure, *Hexamita parva* can be isolated from the urine of affected animals, but this must be examined rapidly after collection.

It is possible to screen urine samples with a practice microscope as movement often leads the observer to the organism in a fresh sample. Urine can often be obtained by gentle manual expression of the bladder between two fingers placed in each of the fossae in front of the hind limbs. Using oil immersion the parasite can usually be seen as a small highly active 'balloon on a string'. Zwart & Truyens (1975) described the parasite as moving fast and in straight lines, often rotating about its long axis. Anterior and posterior flagella may be present, but the two posterior flagella of unequal length are more notable. The parasite measures about 8 μm by 4.5 μm.

**Signs of *Hexamita parva* infection**

- Strongly smelling urine
- Urine dark green or flecked with blood
- Polydipsia
- Anorexia
- Fluid retention (oedema) or weight loss are possible

### Diagnosis

Isolation of *Hexamita* spp. from direct microscopy of urine or other samples. Any animal with one or more of the above symptoms should be screened for the disease.

### Treatment

The treatment is usually metronidazole, although doses of other protozoan active drugs are given later in the section on 'Drugs and dosages' (dimetronidazole and ronidazole).

| Metronidazole (various, e.g. Flagyl suspension, May and Baker) |
|---|
| • 240–260 mg/kg as an oral dose repeated after 14 days (this seems to be the dose of choice).<br>• 160 mg/kg daily for four days and<br>• 35 mg/kg daily for ten days |

### Prognosis

Good if caught early or as a routine screen. Guarded if clinical symptoms, particularly fluid retention, are present.

| A control plan for *Hexamita* spp. infection |
|---|
| • Prevent overcrowding.<br>• Remove faecal and other matter quickly.<br>• Regular disinfection of environment.<br>• Screen colonies and all new arrivals before contact is permitted.<br>• Isolate infected animals at once. |

## BALANTIDIUM (spp.)

A ciliate protozoan organism regularly isolated in domestic tortoises. No specific disease has been attributed to it. It appears to be relatively easy to clear this organism using a single dose of metronidazole at 260 mg/kg.

## AMOEBIASIS

Again of limited significance to the tortoise but it should be noted that snakes, which are highly susceptible to *Entamoeba invadens*, should not be kept in close proximity to tortoises if at all possible and accommodation should be thoroughly disinfected after tortoise use.

## COCCIDIOSIS

Coccidiosis is a problem in the green turtle (Leibovitz *et al.* 1978; Gordon *et al.* 1993).

Jacobson (1994) documents several papers that have identified coccidiosis in tortoises and a recent paper by Jacobson *et al.* (1994b) describes intranuclear coccidiosis in two sick radiated tortoises (*Geochelone radiata*) with symptoms of the infection including nephritis, hepatitis, enteritis and pancreatitis.

The paper by Gordon *et al.* (1993) documents coccidiosis in an epizootic episode in free living green turtles where enteritis and encephalitis were the presenting symptoms. They identify that the problem is not necessarily restricted to turtle farms as previously thought but is also present in the wild population as well.

# A SUGGESTED APPROACH TO DIARRHOEA

Diarrhoea may occur as a condition in its own right or as a symptom of a variety of conditions.

| Possible causative factors | Important details of history |
|---|---|
| • Helminth infections<br>• Protozoan infections<br>• Bacterial infections<br>• Fungal infections<br>• Inappropriate diet<br>• Vitamin deficiency<br>• Antibiotic treatment (sterile gut syndrome)<br>• Chronic debility<br>• *Mycoplasma/Chlamydia* infections<br>• Viral infections | • Recent worming<br>• Recent mixing of groups<br>• Condition of in contact animals<br>• Normal diet<br>• Dietary changes<br>• Previous treatments |

## CLINICAL EXAMINATION

See the section entitled 'Clinical examination'.

## DIAGNOSTIC SAMPLES

Faecal samples should be examined for protozoa (immediate microscopy), faecal egg counts (flotation and microscopy), bacterial culture and sensitivity, and fungal identification (esp. *Candida* spp.).

**A treatment plan for diarrhoea**

- Provide fluids to maintain hydration (traditional rehydration solutions).
- Maintain nutritional status in the face of poor digestion and decreased gut passage time.
- Dietary changes. Increase fibre levels, decrease fructose–sugar levels. This will increase gut passage time, provide faecal bulk and decrease the likelihood of fungal superinfection. Oral kaolin preparations, such as Kaopectate: Upjohn, may also be of use.
- Probiotics (see sterile gut syndrome) to recolonize the gut.
- Prophylactic ketoconazole if fungal superinfection is anticipated.
- Specific treatment related to underlying infections. Anthelmintic, antiprotozoans, antifungals, antibiotics as described in the appropriate sections.

# ANAESTHESIA

## TEMPERATURE

Great care should be taken to maintain the anaesthetized tortoise's body temperature suitably, using a heat pad or hot water bottle. The preferred optimum temperature (POT) for the species concerned would be most suitable otherwise 22°C is normally the recommended anaesthesia temperature and 25°C is the recommended recovery temperature. Variations from this range, particularly below it, can affect the detoxification of anaesthetic agents and other drugs and result in prolonged recovery. Shildiger *et al.* (1993) achieved good results by preheating reptiles to between 25° and 30°C.

## HYDRATION

Fluid therapy both pre-operatively and post-operatively, as described under the heading 'Stomach tubing and oral dosing a tortoise' in the section on 'Handling, injection and feeding techniques', can help in maintaining renal and hepatic function thus maximizing metabolism and excretion of anaesthetic agents and promoting a rapid recovery from anaesthesia.

## INTERMITTENT POSITIVE PRESSURE VENTILATION (IPPV)

This is normally required during a tortoise anaesthetic as tortoises seldom exhibit spontaneous respiration during general anaesthesia. It is not unusual for a chelonian to require assistance with respiration throughout the whole of the anaesthetic period, sometimes the corneal reflex and an ECG trace are the only indication that an anaesthetized tortoise has not expired. In my experience this is often the case when propofol has been used for induction. A pulse oximeter is the ideal method of assessing the required frequency of ventilation but this is not often available in general practice. The rate should mimic the respiration rate of the resting animal, about 10 ventilations per minute are suitable. The inspiratory to expiratory time ratio should be about 1:2. During the recovery phase a tortoise should remain intubated but ventilation can be aided by limb movements. It is normally easy to hear this as it occurs.

## PREMEDICATION

Both atropine sulphate (0.01–0.04 mg/kg) i.m. and acepromazine maleate (0.1–0.5 mg/kg) i.m. have been used in reptiles (Frye 1991). I am unsure as to their efficacy.

## INTUBATION

After appropriate induction. A 3, 4 or larger French gauge Jackson cat catheter (shortened), customized drip tube giving set, large i.v. catheter can all be placed into the trachea. This is achieved by pulling the tongue forward with some protected forceps and inserting the tube into the rima glottidis, which can be found centrally $\frac{2}{3}$ of the way down the tongue. It is usually possible to use ordinary connectors or a shortened 2 ml syringe to link these endotracheal tubes to an Ayres T-piece in order to apply intermittent positive pressure ventilation (IPPV) for the duration of anaesthesia.

## INJECTABLE ANAESTHETICS

Plate 17 shows the intravenous induction of anaesthesia by injection of Saffan into the dorsal venous sinus of the tail of a red-eared terrapin.

| **Alphaxalone/alphadolone** (Saffan: Mallinckrodt) | |
|---|---|
| **Intravenous route** | • 9 mg/kg may be given intravenously (see advice on intravenous injection techniques in the 'Handling, injection and feeding techniques' section). |
| | • This results in an excellent plane of surgical anaesthesia that lasts for 10 or more minutes. I have never had any problems with this agent. It is currently my drug of choice for induction.<br>• It also allows intubation and continuation with a volatile anaesthetic agent. |

| | |
|---|---|
| **Intramuscular route** | • Should i.v. injection not be successful then 15 mg/kg can be given intramuscularly.<br>• The quadriceps mass tends to be the most suitable site for injection.<br>• This tends to have the effect of heavily sedating the tortoise allowing a much smaller dose to be given intravenously to achieve anaesthesia.<br>• Obviously great care must be taken to ensure a fatal overdose is not given if repeated or incremental doses are given. |

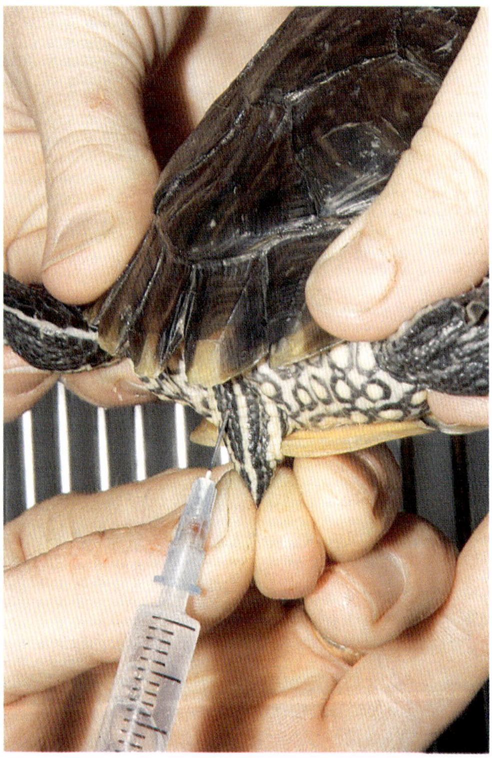

**Plate 17** Intravenous induction of anaesthesia by injection of Saffan: Mallinckrodt into the dorsal venous sinus of the tail of a red-eared terrapin. Take care with intravenous anaesthetic injection as it can be very much slower in onset than with cats and dogs. With agents such as propofol, it can be tempting to give a bit more and a bit more because it doesn't seem to have been particularly effective, only to find the effect appearing five to ten minutes later. Slow, gradual, incremental induction is advised.

| **Propofol** (Rapinovet: Mallinckrodt) |
| --- |
| • This may be given at 1.0–1.4 ml/kg intravenously. Propofol can only be given by the i.v. route.<br>• It results in rapid anaesthesia with a rapid recovery.<br>• Intubation is required for most procedures.<br>• Prolonged periods of apnoea often occur in tortoises anaesthetized with this agent, especially if the patients involved are debilitated. It is not unusual for a tortoise to fail to breathe for the entire surgical procedure, or even 20 minutes or more afterwards. Often it is only the corneal and palpebral blink reflexes that indicate that the animal is still alive (if ECG and pulse oximeter are not available). Whilst this is most alarming at the time I have never seen a tortoise fail to recover if ventilated appropriately, sometimes for up to an hour. The use of a pulse oximeter will help relieve operator anxiety here. My advice is to try not to worry if the tortoise appears apnoic. Carry on as usual and ensure that the patient is ventilated and warm.<br>• Apnoea is more evident when the drug is injected too rapidly as a bolus dose can be reduced by slowly dosing to effect. In my experience the time from dose to effect can be very long, perhaps as much as five minutes, so don't be tempted to give too much too quickly if the propofol does not seem to have worked. Intubate straight after induction. |

## VOLATILE/GASEOUS ANAESTHETICS

| | |
| --- | --- |
| **Halothane** | • Halothane can be used to maintain anaesthesia at 1–2% with oxygen.<br>• This is dependent upon maintaining the animal within its preferred optimum temperature range.<br>• An Ayres T-piece should be used in conjunction with intubation and positive pressure ventilation, as observation of respiratory movements is unreliable.<br>• Tortoises can also be induced with halothane and a 'gas chamber' but compared to induction with Saffan or propofol, this is a crude technique. It is of no use in most Chelonia as they breath-hold. |
| **Isoflurane** | • Probably the best anaesthetic gas for Chelonia and other exotics.<br>• Ex-hospital paediatric 'tec' type machines are available with calibrations for isoflurane, at low cost. The anaesthetic cost is higher than with other volatile anaesthetic agents. |

| | |
|---|---|
| | • Anaesthesia can be maintained at 1–1.5% but this is dependent upon maintaining the animal within its preferred optimum temperature range.<br>• An Ayres T-piece should be used in conjunction with intubation and positive pressure ventilation.<br>• This agent has great advantages in its rapid uneventful recovery and this relates to the very small amount of metabolism (~0.8%) required for this gas.<br>• It is also of great use in animals with compromised hepatic function. |
| **Nitrous oxide** | • This can be used at 2:1 mixture with oxygen and in so doing reduces the amount of volatile anaesthetic by about 25%.<br>• Muscle relaxation is greatly increased and recovery time shortened.<br>• A ten minute period of re-oxygenation is wise before disconnection from the anaesthetic circuit. |
| **Methoxyflurane** | • Used in the same way as halothane but care must be taken with animals suspected of having liver disease or toxaemia.<br>• A very low concentration is adequate. |

## OTHER AGENTS

| | |
|---|---|
| **Ketamine HCl** | • A dissociative psychotropic agent.<br>• It should not be used in animals with suspected renal disease, hepatic disease, dehydration or undiagnosed debilitation as it may prove to be unsafe or even fatal. This is perhaps a product of the time taken to metabolize and detoxify the drug. The main problem would seem to relate to a prolonged and stressful recovery.<br>• A healthy tortoise may be given an i.m. dose of 60–100 mg/kg.<br>• The incidence of reported complications has been greater with higher dosages.<br>• The patient may remain inactive for several hours afterwards or may well continue to make voluntary movements throughout this period.<br>• Personality changes have been reported in other reptiles though this is hard to prove.<br>• Analgesia is questionable when this agent is used alone. Local anaesthetic agents or volatile agents should also be considered. |

| | |
|---|---|
| **Succinylcholine chloride** | • Not a true anaesthetic but a neuromuscular blocking agent with no analgesic properties.<br>• Its use has been advised by Page & Mautino (1990) at a dose of 0.25–1.5 mg/kg but it is only of use in restraint.<br>• Its use in man has declined as it is considered very painful and frightening to the patient. Its use *must* be combined with local or gaseous anaesthesia but it would be very hard to monitor sensation and analgesia in such a patient (pulse oximetry and ECG may be of use in assessing depth of anaesthesia etc.).<br>• Page & Mautino (1990) claim it to be the safest drug available to immobilize tortoises, but insist it be used in the thoracic limb.<br>• This type of drug should not be used in combination with drugs such as aminoglycosides or drugs assumed to be potentially nephrotoxic.<br>• ***It is possible that it is unsuitable for veterinary use in tortoises for the reasons above.*** |
| **Tiletamine/ Zolezepam (Telazol)** | • This has been described at a dose rate of 2 mg/kg by Gould *et al.* (1992) in the red-eared slider, although the specific preparation was not described.<br>• 10–30 μg/kg i.m. seems to be the recommended reptile dose.<br>• Gould *et al.* (1992) intubated and continued surgical anaesthesia using a halothane oxygen mixture and intermittent positive pressure ventilation (IPPV). |
| **Local anaesthesia** | • Lignocaine preparations have been used by local infiltration without adverse effects by many authors and their use has been combined with other agents such as ketamine or gaseous anaesthetics.<br>• The tortoise's legs can be taped inside the carapace in flexion to help immobilize a conscious patient during surgery but this is perhaps crude. |

## COLD NARCOSIS/HYPOTHERMIC ANAESTHESIA

- One of the oldest methods of immobilizing/anaesthetizing reptiles.
- It is not ***advised*** as reptiles which are unable to move because they are chilled may still perceive pain.
- ***I understand it is now illegal to use this form of 'anaesthesia' in the UK.***

## MONITORING AND MAINTENANCE OF ANAESTHESIA

| | |
|---|---|
| **Pulse oximetry and ECG** | • These have been used with encouraging results by the author to effectively monitor pulse heartbeat and respiration.<br>• The probe/sensor can attach to a flap of skin on the proximal hind limb. |
| **Reflexes** | • Withdrawal, palpebral, corneal and 'pain' reflexes are all of use in assessing degree of anaesthesia. It is not unusual for the only positive sign of life to be the corneal blink reflex during anaesthesia. |
| **Intermittent positive pressure ventilation (IPPV)** | • This should always be used, as previously described, where accurate assessment of depth of anaesthesia is not considered possible. |

Plates 18 and 19 show ideal monitoring of anaesthesia in a red-eared terrapin undergoing surgery.

### Ideal monitoring of anaesthesia in a red-eared terrapin undergoing surgery (Plates 18 and 19)

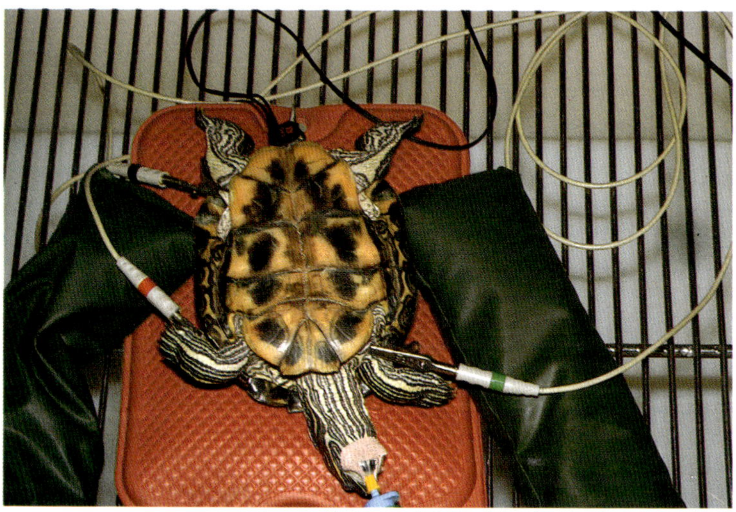

**Plate 18** This tortoise is intubated and being maintained on gaseous anaesthesia (isoflurane) using IPPV. A hot water bottle is used to maintain a warm body temperature. Three ECG leads, connected to two forelimbs and one hind limb, give a reasonable trace and confirm the heart rate. A pulse oximeter sensor has been connected to the tail. This gives a reading that correlates to the degree of oxygenation of the blood and this can be used in order to regulate the frequency of IPPV.

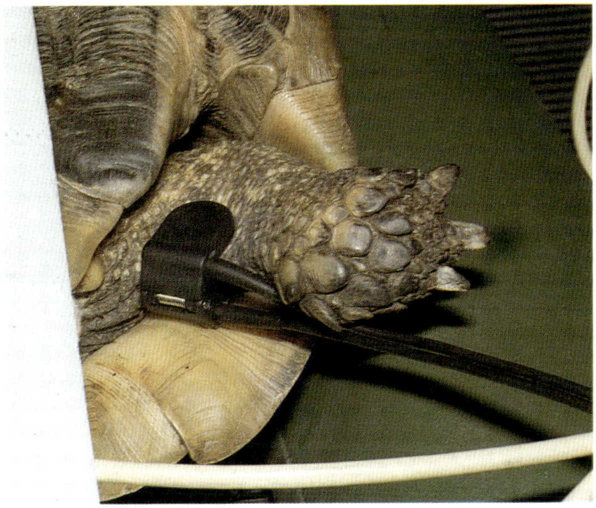

**Plate 19** The sensor for a pulse oximeter is easily connected to a flap of skin of an anaesthetized tortoise. The sensor measures the colour changes in blood that occur with differing levels of oxygenation. As the oxygenation reading falls the tortoise can be ventilated. This results in the reading returning back to a suitable level of oxygenation.

# SURGICAL TECHNIQUES AND SHELL REPAIRS

General anaesthesia using agents such as Saffan or propofol allows a range of surgical procedures to be performed. It is suggested that gut is poorly absorbed in Chelonia, I tend to use PDS (Ethicon). A simple treatment vivarium is an asset during the nursing of sick tortoises (Plate 20).

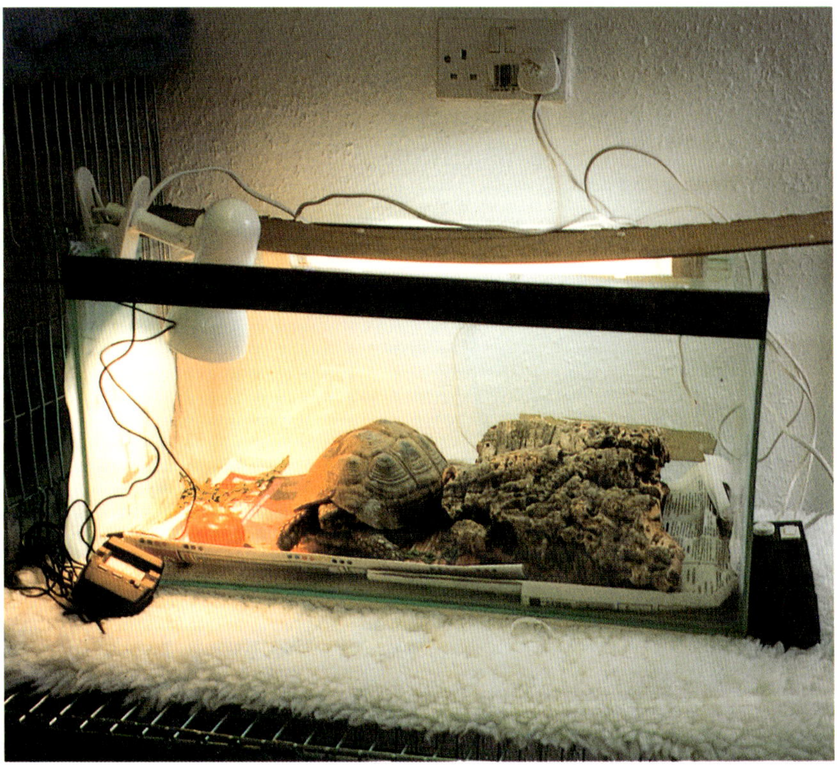

**Plate 20** A simple treatment vivarium is an asset during the nursing of sick tortoises. The vivarium consists of a simple fish tank. A heat and light source is provided by a simple clip-on lamp with a 60W bulb. A true light fluorescent strip is also in operation, although this is not essential if hospitalizing animals for short periods of time only. A digital thermometer is present, in this case with its probe at the warm end of the tank. A large piece of cork provides shelter for food from the heat and relieves boredom. Care must be taken to maintain a suitable humidity.

| Common Chelonian surgical procedures |
|---|
| • Curetting/removal of abscesses<br>• Eye enucleation<br>• Limb amputation<br>• Shell drilling in pneumonia<br>• Amputation of traumatized penis<br>• Coeliotomy (e.g. for egg retention or for foreign body removal)<br>• Shell damage repair |

## CURETTING/REMOVAL OF ABSCESSES

Abscesses can be found in various sites but the ear, limb or a retrobulbar occurrence are common. Two types of abscess are often encountered: inspissated and active.

| Inspissated | Active |
|---|---|
| • These often shell out and do well if left open and well ventilated to heal. | • Culture and sensitivity is often very rewarding. (Often Gram-negative infections.)<br>• Exposure after curettage improves oxygenation and therefore healing.<br>• These can sometimes be sutured if the capsule is also totally excised. |

The surgery is performed under general anaesthesia (Plate 21). Circumscribed, discrete abscesses are completely excised and the tissues sutured to produce first intention healing.

Abscesses involved in other structures, such as those in the ear area, may not be amenable to total excision. Curettes such as those used in orthopaedic surgery may be of value during debridement and if all infected tissue cannot be removed, the surgeon may wish to try to leave the area well-ventilated and allow second intention healing with or without local antibiotics (e.g. gentamicin ointment). Post-operative cleansing and management should be monitored over the following few weeks. It is important to check the oropharynx for extension of an aural abscess into the eustacean tube.

Where particularly resistant organisms with no appropriate antibiotic treatment are encountered and recurrence and cellulitis have occurred,

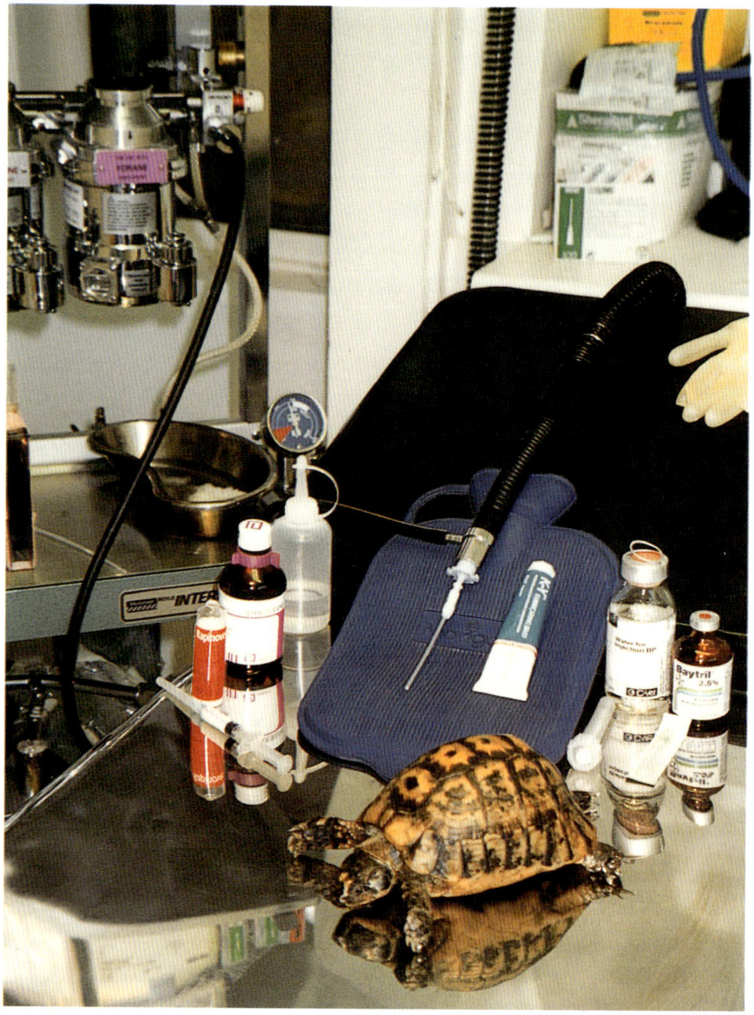

**Plate 21** Anaesthetic and surgical requirements for the treatment of a chronic ear abscess are easily met by most practices. Induction is possible with intravenous propofol or Saffan. Simple urethral catheters can be used to intubate a tortoise and isoflurane or halothane used for maintenance in conjunction with IPPV. A hot water bottle is excellent at maintaining a suitable body temperature.

cryosurgery of the affected area with post-operative exposure/ventilation may prove to be of value.

## EYE ENUCLEATION

This is much as one would expect for any small animal. As the healing process is so much slower in reptiles, these animals are not desutured until after healing has taken place and this is expected to take 4–6 weeks. The eye is removed along with the lid margins. The dead space is closed down and the skin sutured with sheathed nylon or monofilament.

## LIMB AMPUTATION

This may be the treatment of choice for septic arthritis. Wherever possible soft tissues are stripped from the bone and these are used to cover the stump. Just like any other small animal operation, vessels are ligated and skin closure routine. High amputations are always indicated to minimize trauma to any stump. Skin sutures should be removed in 4–6 weeks. See the earlier note regarding Lego® prosthesis when dealing with septic arthritis within the section on 'Bacterial infections'.

## SHELL DRILLING IN PNEUMONIA

- This is a simple technique used in emergencies to swab the dorsally lying lung tissue directly for culture purposes and to facilitate direct application of antibiotics in acute or chronic pneumonias.
- The lesions are located using dorso–ventral and lateral radiographs and a large diameter drill used to penetrate the carapace. It must be remembered that if this is done conscious, then pain may result – the shell is alive!
- A sterile Blu-tac®, or similar, plug may be used to fill the defect between treatments and this can later be repaired with a permanent resin plug, as above, if the pneumonia is controlled. It is essential to maintain integrity of the pleural cavity in order for inspiration to occur, as is the case with mammals. Be careful not to allow foreign material to enter through this hole.
- Take care to ensure that any antibiotic applied directly is suitable. It should be a low irritant preparation suitable for direct application into delicate tissues.

## PENILE AMPUTATION

If seriously traumatized then amputation of a penile prolapse may be the most suitable treatment option (see Plates 22–25). Medical and conservative management is described in the section on 'Captive breeding and reproductive problems' under the heading 'Reproductive considerations in the male tortoise'.

## Surgical removal of a cloacal/penile prolapse (Plates 22–25)

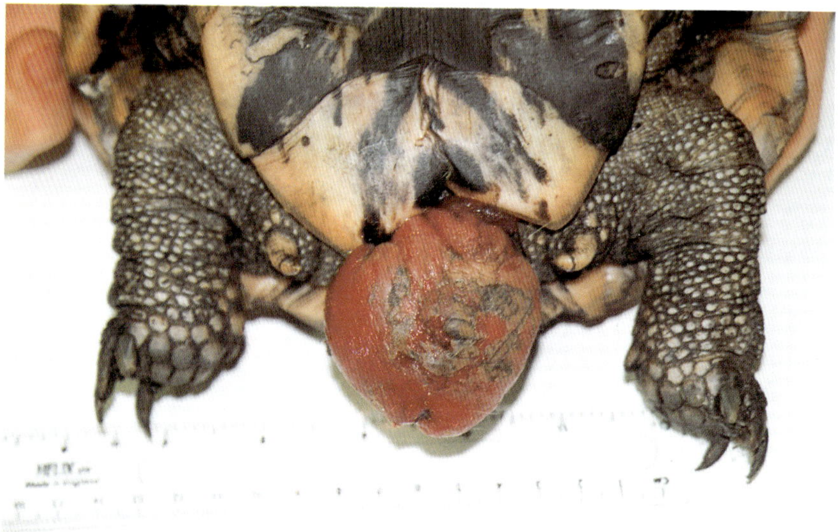

**Plate 22** This large oedematous penile/cloacal prolapse was reduced repeatedly. A purse string suture (PDS: Ethicon) was then used to retain it. Recurrent prolapses over a three week period, in combination with secondary trauma and infection, led to amputation of the prolapse.

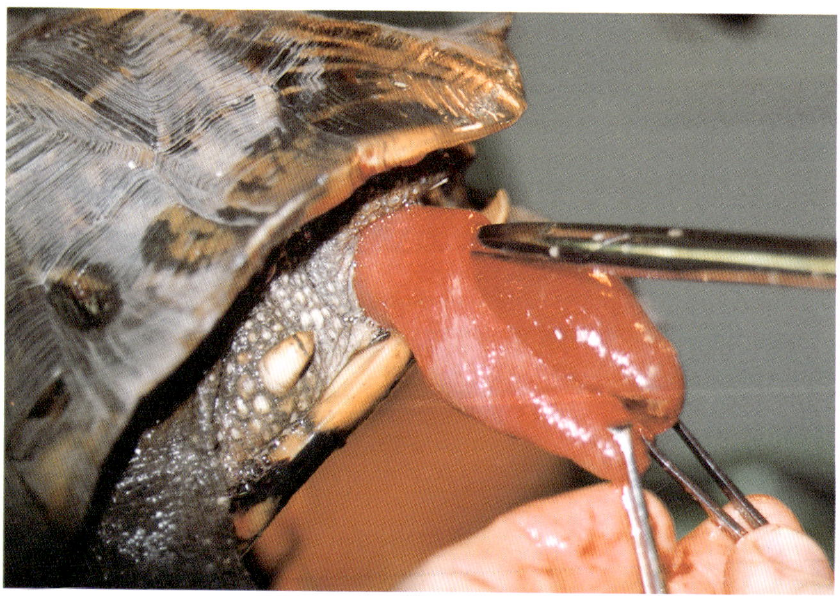

**Plate 23** The area is debrided and prepared suitably for surgery. The prolapse can be easily handled using tissue forceps and the cloacal entrance is identified and protected using blunt ended Mayo scissors.

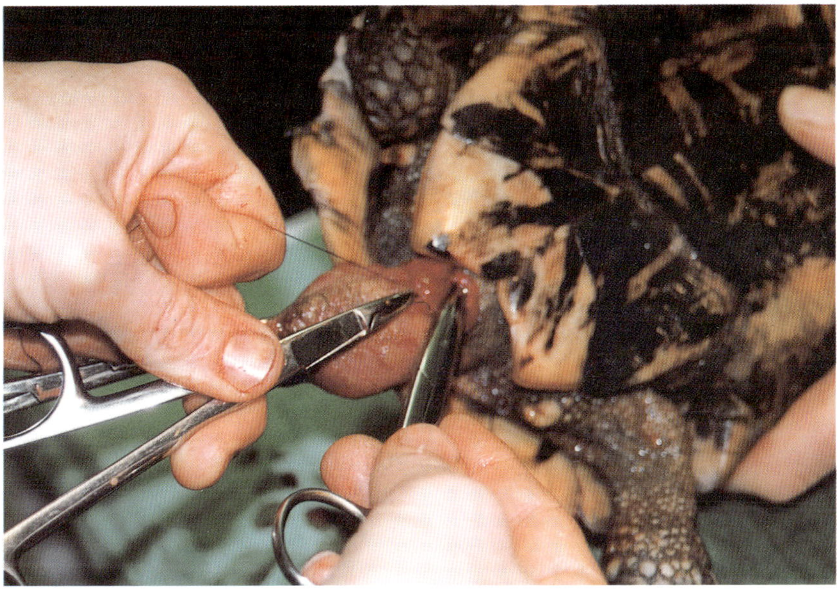

**Plate 24** With Mayo scissors identifying a suitable opening to the cloaca, circumferential mattress sutures (PDS: Ethicon) are made 360 degrees around the prolapse. These ensure haemostasis and seal off the penile/cloacal prolapse.

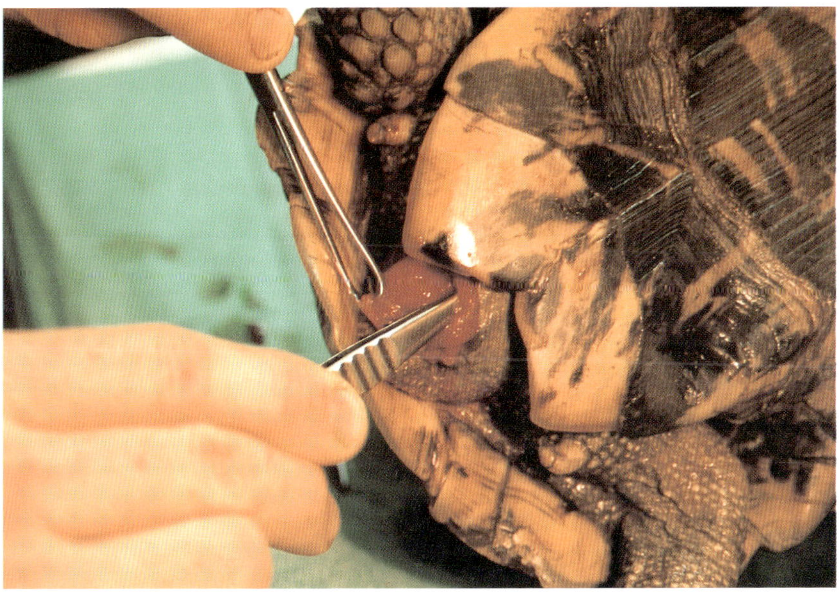

**Plate 25** The prolapse was then removed and the base gently replaced into the cloaca. Urination was not affected but this tortoise will now be infertile. Post-operative enrofloxacin (Baytril: Bayer) was given for ten days using alternate day injections. An uneventful recovery resulted.

**Surgical considerations for penile amputation**

- A vertical mattress suture is placed through healthy proximal penile material, providing haemostasis.
- The devitalized tissue distal to this is then removed by blade, scissors or cautery.
- Post-operative care is minimal but further checks should be made to observe for possible infection.
- The tortoise will become infertile but urination and behaviour will not be affected.

## PLASTRAL COELIOTOMY

Three conditions are regularly treated in this way:

- Intestinal foreign body/obstruction (from radiographic evidence)
- Calculus removal (usually 'cystic' – in the bladder)
- Salpingotomy and removal of impacted ova.

Strict asepsis is essential. Various authors have described surgery performed through a plastral coeliotomy. Such coelial surgery is comparable to traditional mammalian surgery, although it must be remembered that healing time may be longer and this may affect choice of suture material (PDS: Ethicon would appear most suitable). Similarly, the surgeon may wish to use surgical instruments such as spay hooks in order to access and expose viscera.

Plates 26–32 show a plastral coeliotomy to remove an abnormally shaped egg following unsuccessful medical treatment.

**Advice concerning a plastral coeliotomy**

- Radiographs should be taken to help locate, and so avoid, the pelvic girdle.
- The anaesthetized tortoise is placed in dorsal recumbency.
- The patient is maintained at an adequate body temperature.
- Anaesthetic monitoring devices such as ECG/pulse oximetry should be employed if possible.
- The site is prepared as for sterile surgery.
- A high speed orthopaedic burr or plaster cutting circular saw can be used to cut a square flap through the plastron.
- If the flap is removed it is best kept in a physiological solution until it is replaced. It may be possible to rotate the flap leaving one side vascularized and attached. This is desirable.
- The coelomic membrane is exposed by rotation of the flap created.
- The coelomic membrane is incised longitudinally and retracted taking care not to incise bladder tissue.

## Coeliotomy to remove an abnormally shaped egg following unsuccessful medical treatment (Plates 26–32)

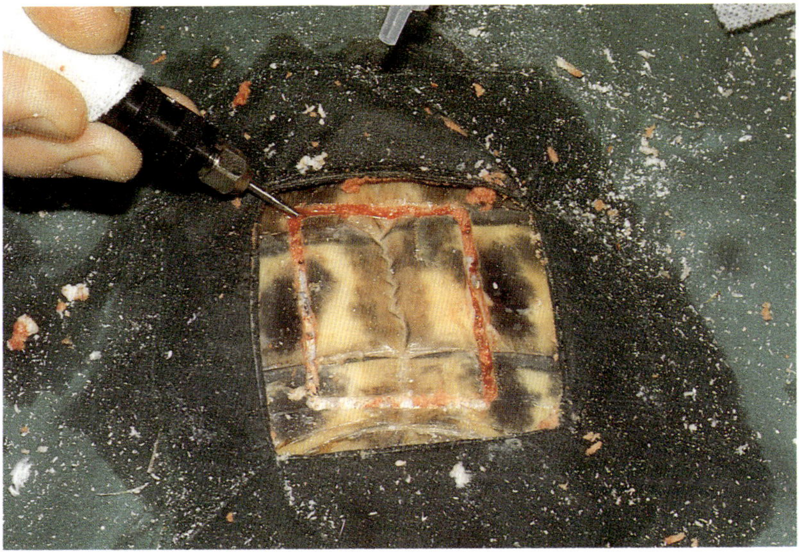

**Plate 26** After taking radiographs of the tortoise to locate the pelvic girdle, the site of coeliotomy is marked out on the plastron of the anaesthetized turtle. The turtle is in dorsal recumbency and the site has been prepared for surgery. A high speed orthopaedic burr is used to cut a flap in the plastron. The cranial flap attachment is preserved in order to maintain a blood supply to the shell tissue. A burr is messy and frequent flushing with sterile saline is required.

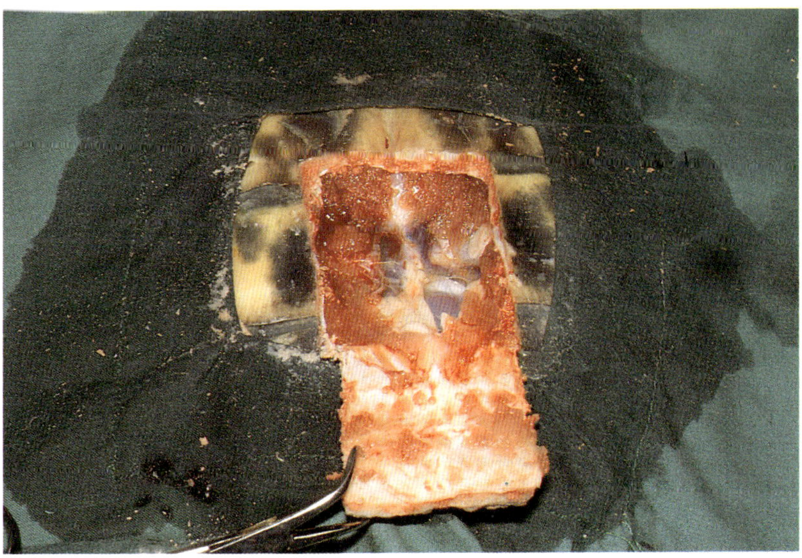

**Plate 27** The flap created is reflected to reveal the coelomic membrane. Take care not to incise bladder tissue when entering the coelomic cavity.

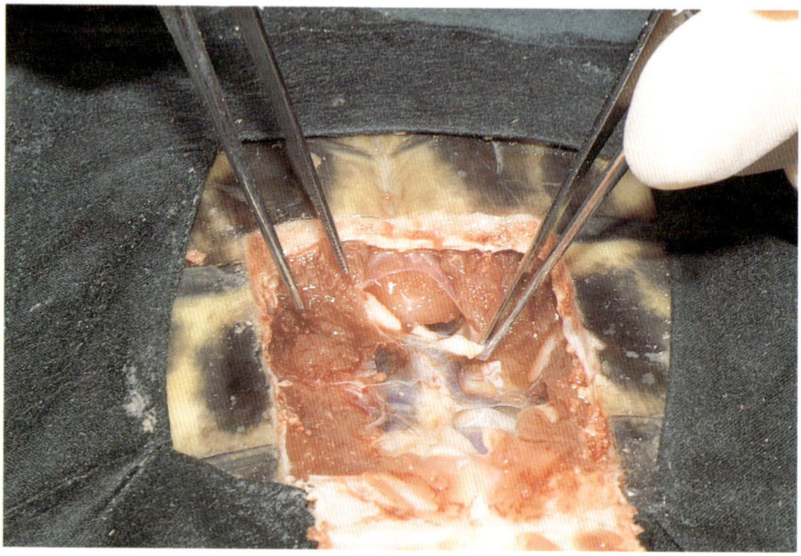

**Plate 28** The coelomic membrane is carefully incised.

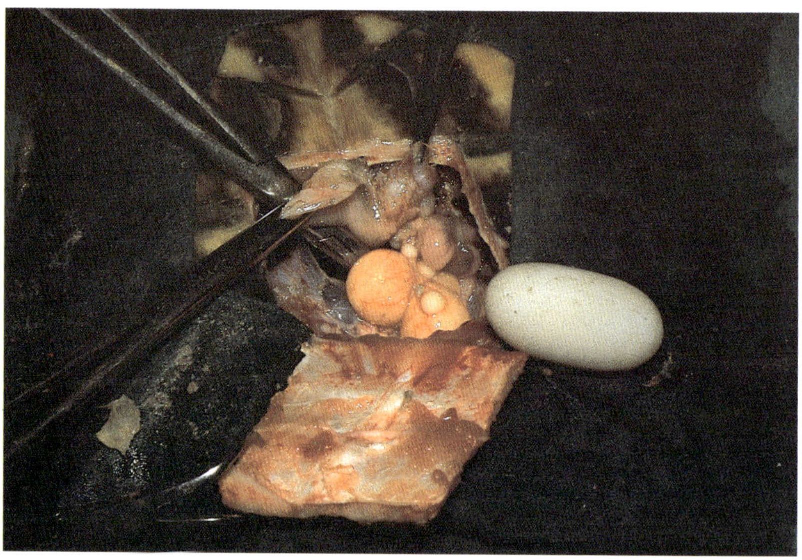

**Plate 29** The abnormal egg is located and removed. Fine PDS (Ethicon) is used for internal suturing.

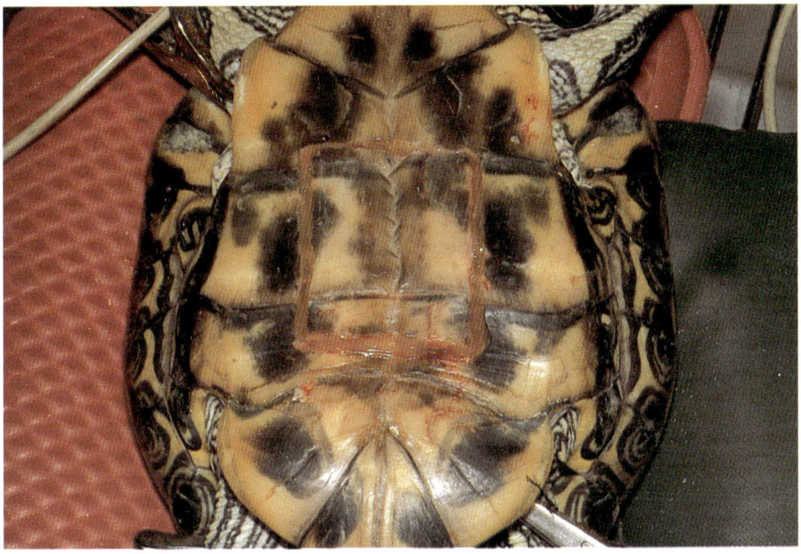

**Plate 30** After closing the coelomic membrane the flap is replaced and a water soluble ointment (K-Y Jelly: Johnson & Johnson) used to fill the crevices. This prevents resin filling the space, which would result in a non-union of the flap.

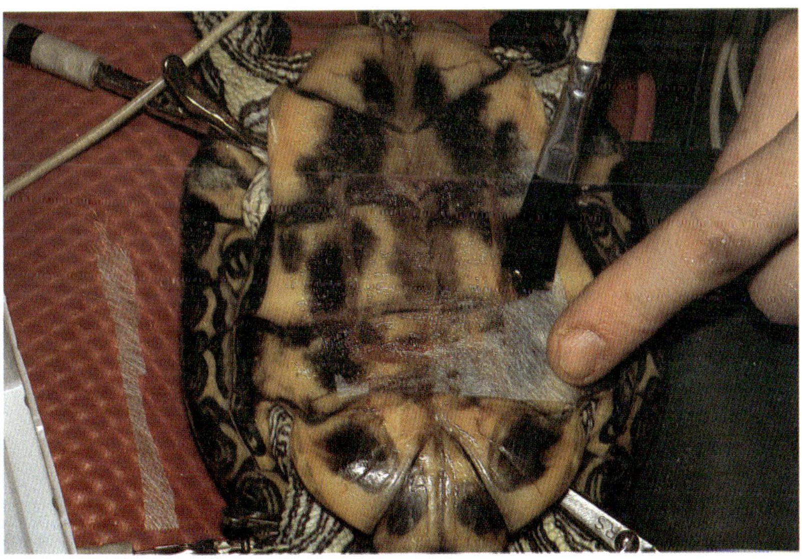

**Plate 31** Fibreglass matting is autoclavable and can be combined with a suitable resin to make good the defect created by the flap.

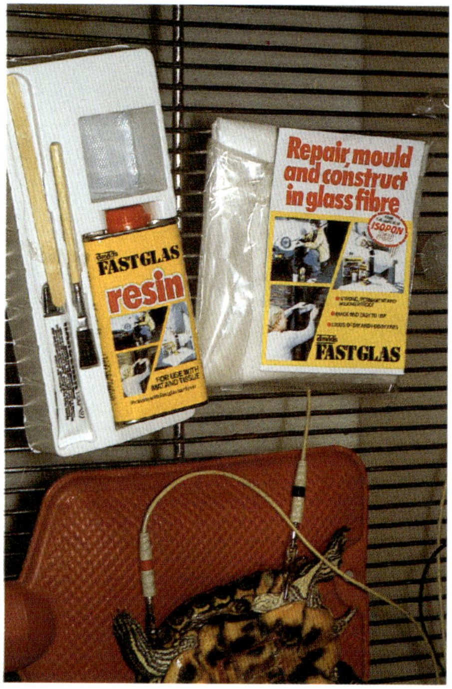


**Plate 32** An example of a resin suitable for coeliotomy closure.

**Advice concerning coeliotomy closure**

- After the coelomic surgery is performed the coelomic membrane is sutured with an absorbable material (e.g. PDS: Ethicon or Vicryl: Ethicon).
- The flap is replaced into the plastral defect. It is important that resin material used in sealing the coeliotomy site is not allowed to fill the fissure between the flap and intact plastron, as this will result in a non-union. Several authors advise filling this fissure with a water-soluble material (e.g. K-Y Jelly: Johnson & Johnson) or perhaps an antibiotic ointment (e.g. gentamicin) before application of resin material.
- The flap and surrounding plastral area are covered in an epoxy resin-like material with polymer added (e.g. methyl methacrylate, dental cement, bone cement, car repair epoxy resin, or similar). It may be beneficial to roughen the site prior to application.
- The flap is adhered to a fibreglass cloth, which may be autoclaved, using a resin material.
- This in turn is adhered to the plastral shell surrounding the coeliotomy site with the resin material. This supports the flap and fixes it in place.
- The defect is then covered in several more layers of resin material and the temperature of the setting material monitored (the reaction is exothermic).

## NON-PLASTRAL COELIOTOMY

Coeliotomy for exposure of the intestine has been described through an alternative soft tissue approach by Britanian (1984) and later by Gould *et al.* (1992) in the red-eared slider (terrapin). These authors used a soft tissue approach through an area just cranial to the hind limb. A spay-hook can be used to expose intestine and the successful removal of an intestinal foreign body has been performed. The muscle closure used PDS (Ethicon) and the skin used nylon sutures. The technique has not been described in the Mediterranean tortoise but anatomical similarities may make similar surgery possible.

## SHELL DAMAGE REPAIR

Several texts have large chapters describing the repair of shell damage, back deformities and fractures, e.g. Frye (1991) and Harvey & Orr (1990) and further information and advice can be found here.

Traumatic shell injuries are common in tortoises (Plate 33). Traumatic injuries caused by boat propellers are common in young turtles that feed close to the water surface (Plate 34).

| | |
|---|---|
| **Conservative treatment** | • Whilst I have made various attempts at repair of shell damage due to trauma from such things as hover-type lawnmowers, persistent gnawing/ chewing by dogs, crush injuries etc., the majority of such injuries once infected appear to do very well if managed conservatively. Initial debridement of injuries should be performed and as time progresses, bandaging the area with a pre-shaped dressing such as Melolin: Smith & Nephew using zinc oxide tape over antibiotic ointment, such as Genticin: Roche, if required. Dermisol: SmithKline Beecham and Aserbine: Forley are also effective as debriding agents.<br>• Such cases tend to do very well if clients participate and facilitate treatment. Healing will take in the region of 1–2 years and overwintering will be essential during this period. Regular consultations fortnightly to monthly will monitor progress. |

| | |
|---|---|
| **Surgical treatment** | • A fractured or surgically opened shell is repaired using epoxy resins much as described previously. If trauma is the cause, devascularized and heavily infected fragments must be discarded. A defect can sometimes be covered with epoxy impregnated fibreglass. Bone will bridge defects after 1–2 years depending on their size. Care must be taken not to seal up an infected site if the lesion is old. It may be wiser to treat such lesions conservatively.<br>• The area is prepared aseptically. The fragment and neighbouring tissue are painted in a five minute epoxy resin or other material as suggested in the closure of a coeliotomy. Care is taken not to allow any fissures to collect the resin (by pre-filling them with antibiotic ointment/K-Y Jelly: Johnson & Johnson). A preformed sheet of fibreglass is placed over the reduced fracture. Further layers of both resin and fibreglass are applied as required. The fibreglass should extend 1.5–3.0 cm beyond the defect. Autoclaving the fibreglass helps to prevent wound infections.<br>• Layers should be applied one at a time and the heat allowed to dissipate prior to applying the next layer.<br>• Occasionally interfragmentary wiring and plating are required. This is particularly true of plastral fractures that experience great tension. Small Kirshner wires/Arthrowires and even small ASIF/non-ASIF plates have a place here.<br>• Healing may take 1–2 years so any implants or restrictive plastics may require removal/replacing if growth is hindered. |

**Plate 33** (opposite) Traumatic shell injuries are common. (a) An infected dog bite injury that involved the caudal shell and the underlying pelvic muscle mass. There were also traumatic injuries to the cloacal entrance and cranial carapace. (b) The wounds were repeatedly cleared of necrotic tissue and daily fluids and enrofloxacin administered. A Pevidine (C-Vet) soaked swab can be used to fill the shell defect until healthy granulation tissue is present. A plastic or fibreglass plug can then cover the area, or it can be left to heal naturally over several weeks and months.

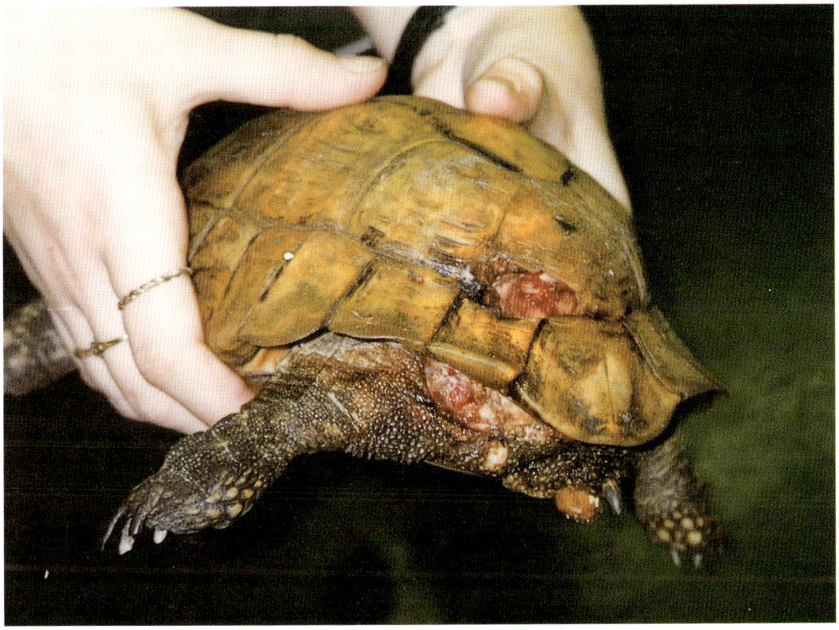

(a)

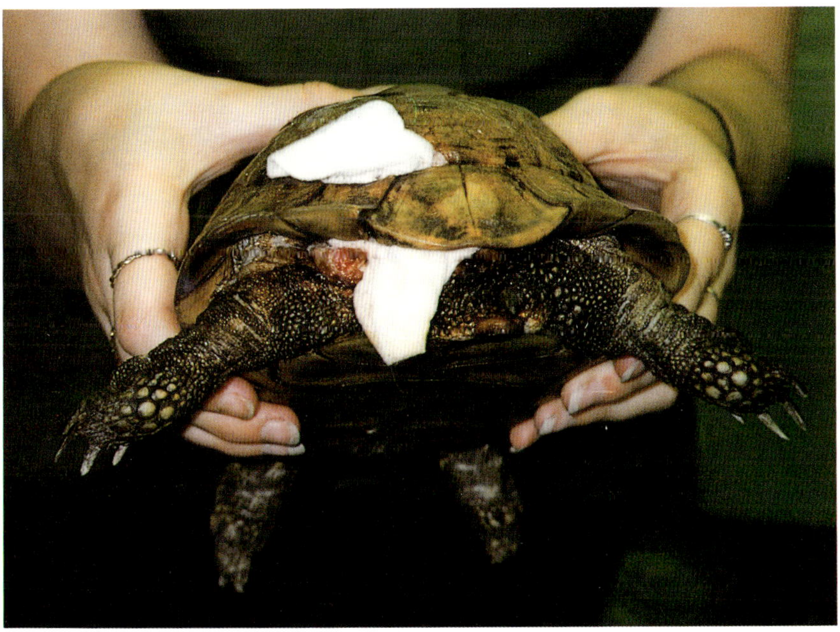

(b)

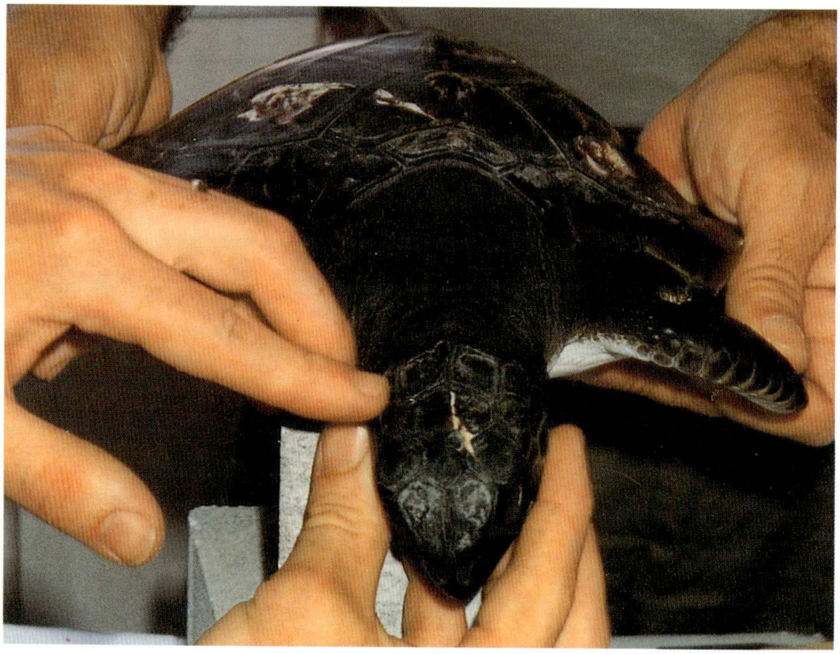

(a)

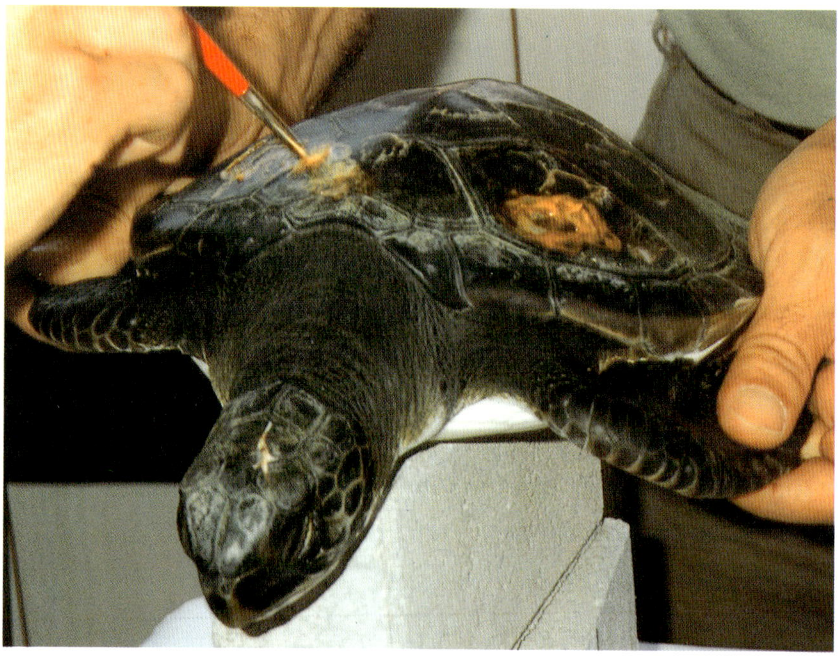

(b)

## MANAGEMENT OF OTHER ACUTE TRAUMA

| | |
|---|---|
| **Burns** | • Normally managed by continued dressing, e.g. Melolin: Smith & Nephew bandaged over a suitable cream (Genticin: Roche/Aserbine: Forley/Dermisol: SmithKline Beecham) |
| **Limb fracture** | • Repair is extrapolated from other species.<br>• Internal fixation is rare, but possible (e.g. i.m. pin).<br>• External fixation techniques include support via plaster/Hexalite (Alfred Cox Surgical Ltd)/ synthetic cast or taping in the affected limb to immobilize it. |

## EXTERNAL CARE OF TORTOISES

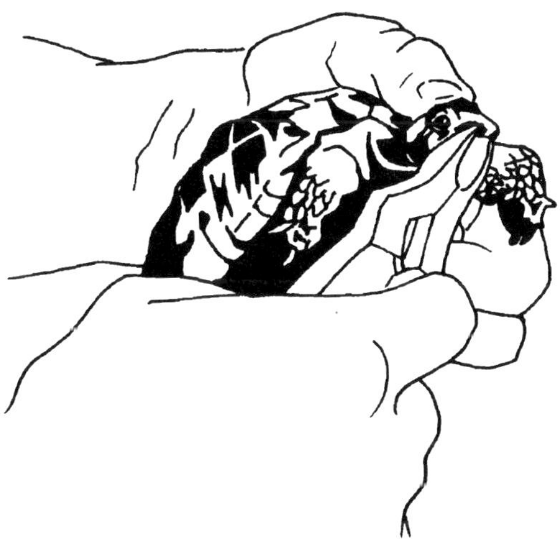

**Fig. 21** Clipping a tortoise's beak. Ordinary nail clippers can be used to remove large amounts of horn and emery boards or nail files can be used to smooth this afterwards.

---

**Plate 34** (opposite) Traumatic injuries caused by boat propellers are common in young turtles that feed close to the water surface. (a) This young green turtle (*Chelonia mydas*) was treated for propeller damage to its skull and carapace. (b) The injuries were debrided and loose material removed with a scalpel. A paint brush was used to clean those areas with a povidone-iodine solution on a twice daily basis. The turtle was kept in an isolation tank and observed for infection during the healing period. Water quality was maintained throughout this time.

| | |
|---|---|
| **Clipping beaks** (Fig. 21) | • Beaks that become overgrown will interfere with prehension.<br>• They can be trimmed cautiously with nail clippers.<br>• They can be filed with nail files/emery boards.<br>• They can be abraded by providing cuttlefish etc. to chew on. |
| **Clipping claws** | • Only really required if an abrasive substrate is not present.<br>• The technique is similar to that used with the cat or dog. |
| **Shell care** | • Shell drilling for tethering is now illegal.<br>• Regular cleaning rather than oiling is advised.<br>• Povidone-iodine solutions are suitable. |

# RADIOGRAPHY

Radiography can help in the specific assessment of disease and in the assessment of its severity. The facilities available will limit the quality of radiographs produced, but even the minimum of equipment can result in diagnostic quality radiographs.

The following is intended as a guide. Alter settings to compensate for different screens, focal distances, tortoise sizes and power of machine.

## STANDARD RADIOGRAPHIC VIEWS

The main body of a tortoise can be examined comprehensively by the use of three views taken at right angles. These are well-shown in Lee (1989/90). Other authors such as Rübel *et al.* (1991), Frye (1991) and Jackson & Sainsbury (1992) also cover the subject.

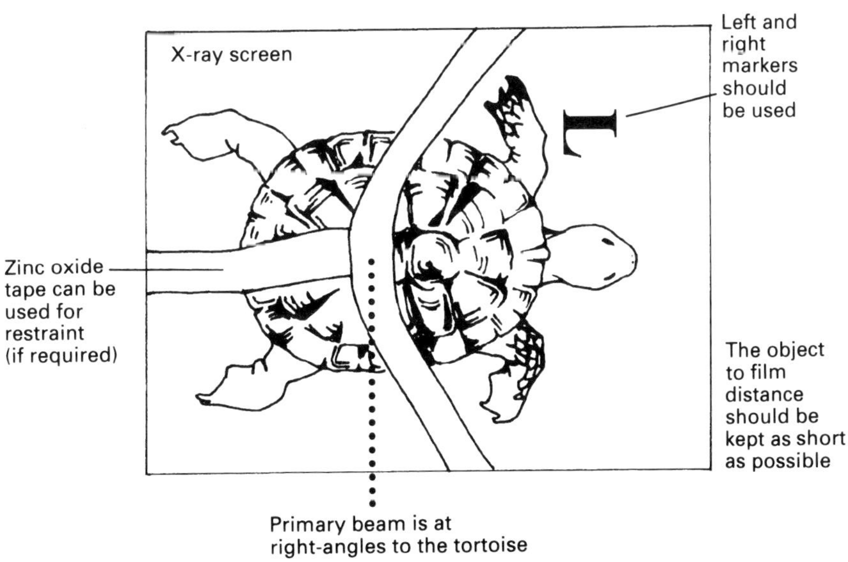


**Fig. 22** The dorso–ventral radiographic view.

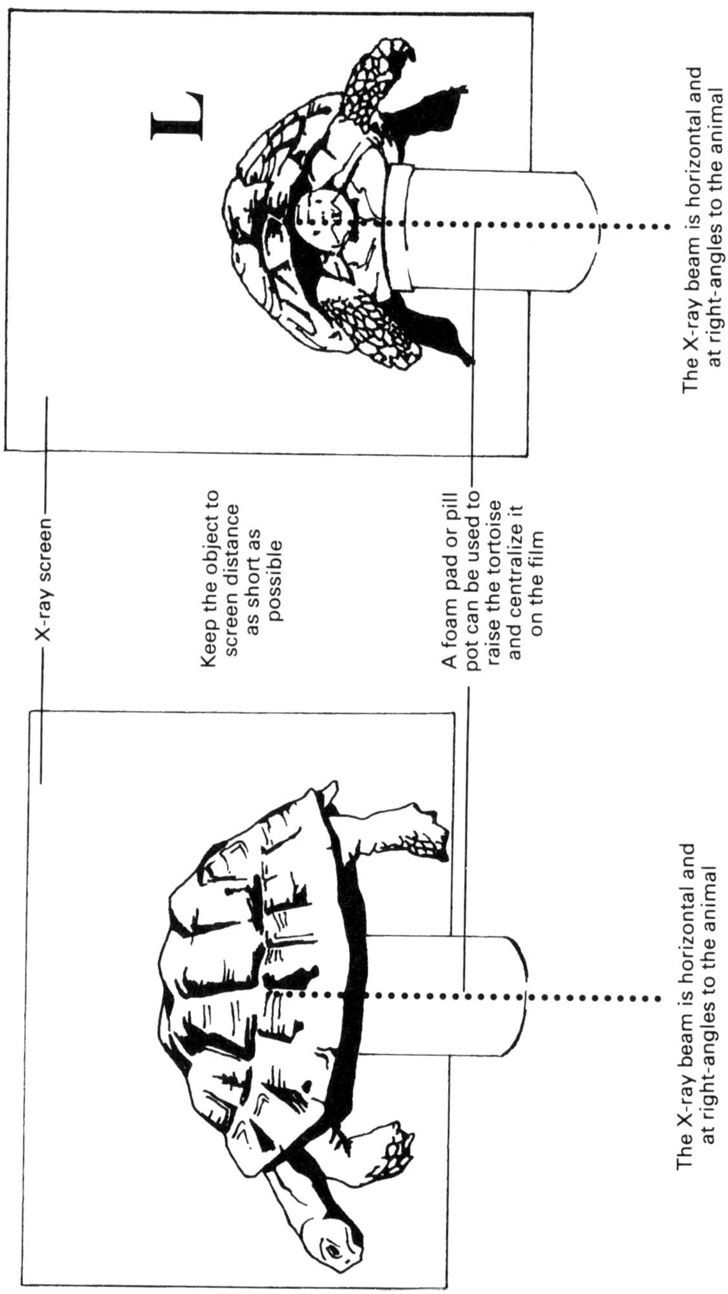


**Fig. 23** The lateral radiographic view.

**Fig.; 24** The cranio–caudal radiographic view.

| | |
|---|---|
| **Dorso–ventral view** (Fig. 22) | This view can be used to examine some visceral organs, the skeletal system and for contrast studies of the digestive system. A vertical beam at right angles to the animal is used (left and right markers should be used). |
| **Lateral view** (Fig. 23) | Once again useful in examining the lung fields. If the beam cannot be rotated to the horizontal the weight of viscera and resulting displacement will make views of a tortoise on its side difficult to interpret. |
| **Cranio–caudal view** (Fig. 24) | This is of use in assessing the lung fields (use left and right markers). |

## EXPOSURE FACTORS

- The mAs should utilize as short an exposure as possible, in order to minimize blur from movement.
- In order to keep the mA s short, as high an mA as is suitable, and available, will result in the shortest exposure time at a given kV.
- The focal distance can be as close as 70 cm using intensifying screens. But if non-screen film or 'Lo-close' film is being used this may need to be increased to about 91 cm.
- High resolution intensifying screens are of great use.
- For a 750 g tortoise measuring 11.5 cm width and 7.5 cm depth exposure factors are given by Jackson & Fasal (1981):

| View | kV | mAs | Focus-film distance | Screen |
|---|---|---|---|---|
| DV | 60 | 10 | 91 cm | fine |
| Lateral | 70 | 16 | 91 cm | fine |

- Fast and standard screens can be used with a static grid or a Potter-Bucky to increase definition.
- Using non-screen film the exposure factors vary with the region under investigation. Jackson & Fasal (1981) suggest 65 kV, 20 mA s at 91 cm. Dental film can be placed between the limb and shell. If the head is under particular examination, dorsal recumbency may be used (Fig. 25).
- 'Lo-Dose' film is not usually available in general practice but Du Pont

Cronex film and Du Pont 2T screens were used at 24 kV, 25 mA and 0.75 s by Jackson & Fasal (1981).

- It is suggested that the operator record successful settings, screens, distances, views and size of animal with their own equipment, as these values are given as a guide.

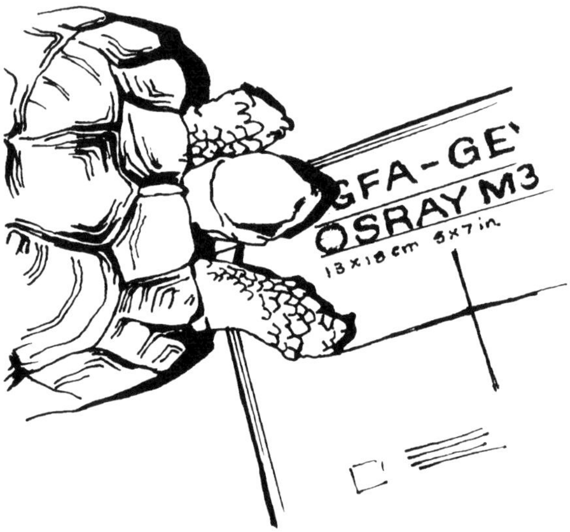


**Fig. 25** The head and limbs expose well on non-screen film.

## RESTRAINT DURING RADIOGRAPHY

It is possible to take radiographs of debilitated, severely ill or well-behaved animals with virtually no restraint at all. Moderate restraint can be provided by zinc oxide tape or adhesive tape and application is reasonably quick. If more energetic animals are under examination then general anaesthesia may be used.

## FURTHER TECHNIQUES

As veterinary science advances, more and more is being made of human diagnostic equipment. The *BSAVA Manual of Reptiles* has a detailed section by Jackson & Sainsbury (1992) on the use of computerized tomography (CT), magnetic resonance imaging (MRI) and ultrasonography of the tortoise. This is also discussed by Frye (1991). The ultrasound 'windows' of the tortoise are explored by Penrinck *et al.* (1991). Ultrasonography is a non-ionizing method of reproductive scanning in Chelonia.

## CONTRAST RADIOGRAPHY

Barium sulphate can be used to outline the stomach and intestines of chelonians. A dose of $20\,cm^3/kg$ bodyweight is suggested. A double contrast technique can be employed by carefully stomach tubing a ***small*** volume of air ($< 15\,cm^3$). Passage time for barium sulphate can be very slow, 24–40 days. It is also affected by temperature and concurrent gastrointestinal disease.

| Notes on radiographic interpretation | |
|---|---|
| **Nutritional osteodystrophy** | Radiography can be used to assess the degree of decalcification of the plastron and carapace. The axillary and inguinal regions are of use here as these show the changes readily. |
| **Pneumonia** | In order to ascertain the extent and location of a pneumonia. Views can be used to locate sites for swabbing and culture/sensitivity. Dorso–ventral lateral, and antero–posterior films with left and right markers should be taken. One or both lung fields may be affected. Radiography is the most important diagnostic technique with pneumonia. |
| **Infectious osteolysis** | Radiography can be used to determine the extent of the problem and to locate a site for amputation should this be required. |
| **Limb fracture/ limb dislocation** | Lesions are easily located if left and right markers are used. Non-screen film may be of use. |
| **Shell fracture** | Skyline views may help visualization and identification of fragments. |
| **Egg retention** | Gravid females retaining eggs will often show a deformed or enlarged egg in the pelvic inlet preventing oviposition. Egg diameter can be measured and compared to pelvic canal diameter. |
| **Calculi** | This can be a cause of egg retention or a problem in its own right. Calculi may occur in the bladder or cloaca. |
| **Foreign body/ intestinal obstruction** | Though uncommon, large amounts of gas tend to be seen and sometimes the foreign body is visualized. Wood screws, coal, and plastic tubing introduced by the client have been recorded. Contrast radiography may be of use. |
| **Oedema** | Antero–posterior views have been used by experienced clinicians. |

# LABORATORY TESTS AND SUITABLE SAMPLES

| Sample | Advice regarding suitable tests |
|---|---|
| **Urine** | This can be used to diagnose cloacal infections. Fresh samples may demonstrate the mobile protozoan *Hexamitas* sp. should it be present. Identification of *Hexamitas* is described elsewhere. Tortoises fed inappropriate diets may demonstrate an excess of glucose in the urine, e.g. milk.<br><br>Urine can often be obtained by gently applying bilateral pressure on the bladder using one finger in each fossa anterior to the hind limbs. |
| **Faeces** | This can be of use in the diagnosis of helminthiasis by faecal egg counts, sterile gut syndrome by consistency, bacterial and possibly protozoan problems by culture. |
| **Swab or aspirate** | As previously discussed routine culture and sensitivity tests are of great use in the tortoise as resistance to antibiotics is perhaps more common than sensitivity. |

## BLOOD SAMPLES

Routine blood screens are of great use in the tortoise, though limited normal values are available. Some laboratories that deal with Chelonia on a regular basis have their own 'normal' range of biochemistry and haematology results for Chelonia but these are, to some extent, specific to the laboratory concerned. It is wise to contact these organizations directly to see what samples are required. Similarly some biochemistry and haematology analysers available in general practice quote values for reptiles such as tortoises. They can also be used to give 'qualitative' results if normal values are unavailable.

Grange Laboratories – PO Box 4, Wetherby, LS22 4ZR – (personal communication, 1993) have kindly supplied the following results as their 'normal' range. The results are derived from more than 100 Chelonia tested. They offer a 'Tortoise Profile' as may other similar laboratories (species are not specified). These figures compare favourably to those of Frye (1991) and Cooper & Beynon (1991).

Grange Laboratories have strongly advised using *heparinized* samples only as it is their experience that the incidence of haemolysis with EDTA samples is very high.

| **Full blood count** | **Normal range** | **Units** |
|---|---|---|
| Red cells | 5.5–8.5 | $\times 10^9$/l |
| Haemoglobin (Hb) | 12.0–18.0 | g/dl |
| Packed cell volume (PCV) | 0.32–0.55 | l/l |
| Mean corpuscular volume (MCV) | 59.0–77.0 | fl |
| Mean corpuscular haemoglobin concentration (MCHC) | 30.0–36.0 | g/dl |
| Mean corpuscular haemoglobin (MCH) | 20.0–26.0 | pg |
| White cells | 06.0–15.0 | $\times 10^9$/l |
| Lymphocytes | 0.50–4.80 | $\times 10^9$/l |
| Monocytes | 0.00–0.60 | $\times 10^9$/l |
| Eosinophils | 0.05–0.60 | $\times 10^9$/l |
| Basophils | 0.00–0.15 | $\times 10^9$/l |

| **Biochemistry** | **Normal range** | **Units** |
|---|---|---|
| Total protein | 55.0–75.0 | g/l |
| Albumin | 25.0–41.0 | g/l |
| Globulin | 20.0–45.0 | g/l |
| AG ratio | 0.60–1.50 | n/a |
| Urea | 02.5–6.70 | mmol/l |
| Creatinine | 20.0–150 | mmol/l |
| ALT @ 37°C | 05.0–60.0 | IU/l |
| ALP @ 37°C | <130 | IU/l |
| GGT @ 37°C | 0.10–9.00 | IU/l |
| AST @ 37°C | 10.0–50.0 | IU/l |
| LDH @ 37°C | 50.0–250 | IU/l |
| Uric acid | 10.0–100 | μmol/l |

- Urea levels are very high post-hibernation and very low pre-hibernation. The time of year is therefore important.
- Urea levels lie between 0 and 200 mmol/l. Values above 18 mmol/l may indicate a possible nephritis or impaired renal function.

- Blood glucose is usually about 10 mmol/l post-hibernation 1.4 mmol/l pre-hibernation.
- PCV is usually about 0.34 post-hibernation 0.28 pre-hibernation.
- Red cell (RBC) count is usually 8.0–9.0 $\times$ $10^9$/l post-hibernation and about 6.0–7.0 $\times$ $10^9$/l pre-hibernation.
- Amongst other things these values reflect hydration.

# CAPTIVE BREEDING AND REPRODUCTIVE PROBLEMS

In view of the legislation affecting the importation of certain species of Chelonia and the threat mankind now poses to these animals, the veterinary profession is obliged to actively encourage responsible breeding wherever possible. Detailed texts on the breeding of tortoises are easily available (e.g. Highfield 1990) and many of the organizations listed at the end of this book will willingly give advice on this subject. Details relating to specific mating and incubation procedures are best obtained from these texts.

Sexual maturity is generally reached at about 15 years of age under natural conditions in most species, but this is greatly influenced by rate of growth and size. Some captive-bred tortoises become sexually active at a very early age; males have been known to mate successfully at four years of age. Females typically attain maturity later than males.

## SEXING TORTOISES

- Mature males have longer tails than females.
- The plastron of males is usually curved or indented.
- Adult males are usually smaller than females.

The typical clutch density of most Mediterranean tortoises is between 4–10 eggs, but this varies considerably between species and subspecies. *Testudo hermanni* (the western population of Hermann's tortoise, inhabiting France and Italy) have a typical clutch density of only three eggs for example, whilst the eastern subspecies *T. h. boettgeri* typically lays clutches of between 6–10 eggs. Egg sizes also vary greatly between various species and subspecies. Two or more clutches per year are possible.

Incubation temperatures play a significant role in determining the sex of the resulting hatchlings. These will vary with species. Incubation humidity and other conditions are best determined by reference to texts describing the natural behaviour of the species concerned.

| Temperature | Result |
|---|---|
| <26° | Eggs usually die |
| 26–29.5°C | All male offspring 74–140 days |
| 30–31.5°C | Mixed offspring |
| 32–34°C | All female offspring 60–75 days |
| >34°C | Deformed hatchlings |

Eggs can be transilluminated using a bright light to see if the yolk has settled but this is not 100% reliable as an indication of fertility. Similarly eggs which are infertile tend to dry out and hence are lighter.

## REPRODUCTIVE CONSIDERATIONS IN THE MALE TORTOISE

### Penile prolapse (Phimosis)

Various factors contribute to this condition, including:

- nutritional osteodystrophy
- bacterial infections
- parasitic infections
- fungal infections
- constipation
- general debility
- libido.

If a predisposing condition is suspected it should be investigated and treated if possible.

#### *Treatment*

- Recent prolapses can usually be reduced if ample lubrication is provided (K-Y Jelly: Johnson & Johnson, obstetric lubricant, etc.).
- The prolapse should be cleaned with a suitable disinfectant solution such as dilute povidone-iodine solution (Pevidine: C-Vet).
- If the prolapse is not yet traumatized but too engorged to reduce, then osmotic agents may help reduce its size. Glycerine, honey and sucrose have been used with varying success.
- The prolapse will generally require a purse-string suture (using PDS: Ethicon) to temporarily hold it in place. The suture is placed around the cloacal aperture and removed a few days later.

- Traumatized, necrotic, or infected prolapses may require amputation under general anaesthesia. This is described in the section on 'Surgical techniques and shell repairs'.

## MALE AGGRESSION

With some variations between species, male tortoises exhibit dramatic aggression during warm summer days. It seems worth commenting that dominant animals can inflict considerable damage on smaller, weaker males and vulnerable females and should be observed closely and even separated from others if required. The number of animals in a colony will also be significant here as keeping a dominant male with a less aggressive one will result in intensive bullying, whereas an increased number of weaker males and females will dilute this aggression and spread out any damage. Observation is essential.

## REPRODUCTIVE CONSIDERATIONS IN THE FEMALE TORTOISE

The most common reproductive problem in the female tortoise requiring veterinary attention is egg retention. Egg retention need not be an anatomical problem with an obstructive cause. The environment of a tortoise is a very important factor in the induction of oviposition, or egg laying (see Plate 35).

It is important to note the duration of symptoms that have led to a diagnosis of egg retention (see Plate 36). It is not uncommon to diagnose the problem as a result of complications such as egg peritonitis where the tortoise is already seriously ill. Examination of cloacal discharges and perhaps even transabdominal aspiration of fluid may indicate that egg peritonitis is present. This will result in a very poor prognosis at the outset of treatment and this should be explained to the client, particularly if a coeliotomy is to be attempted.

## MANAGEMENT OF EGG RETENTION

### Diagnosis

**Ballottement:** Two fingers can be inserted into the fossae anterior to the hind limbs and the tortoise rocked gently from side to side. This allows mineralized ova to be felt. It may also assist in the detection of cloacal or urinary calculi impeding the progress of oviposition.

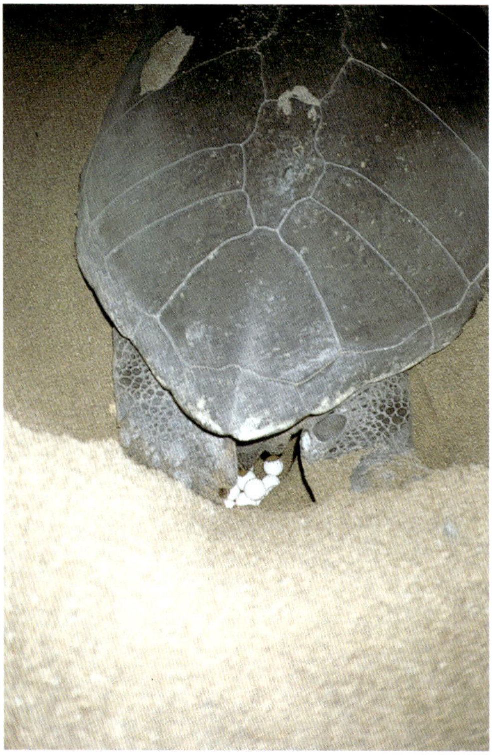

**Plate 35** Oviposition in Chelonia is influenced by environment and instinct. This green turtle (*Chelonia mydas*) has returned to the beach where it hatched many years ago. The egg laying ritual in the green turtle often takes as long as six or seven hours. If animals are disturbed before a suitable nest site is located they often abort egg laying and jettison their eggs in the sea. The massive development of beach resorts over the past 30 years is precipitating the extinction of most turtle species as the beaches where turtles used to lay are no longer suitable. This photograph was taken as part of a conservation project protecting laying turtles in Greek Cyprus.

**Radiography:** This is an essential aid to diagnosis. Evidence from such a radiograph can be used to decide whether the case should be managed medically or surgically at the start.

**A well-taken dorso–ventral radiograph can be used to assess**

- Gravidity
- Size of pelvic canal/opening
- Size of coelomic eggs
- Egg abnormalities
- Obstructive calculi

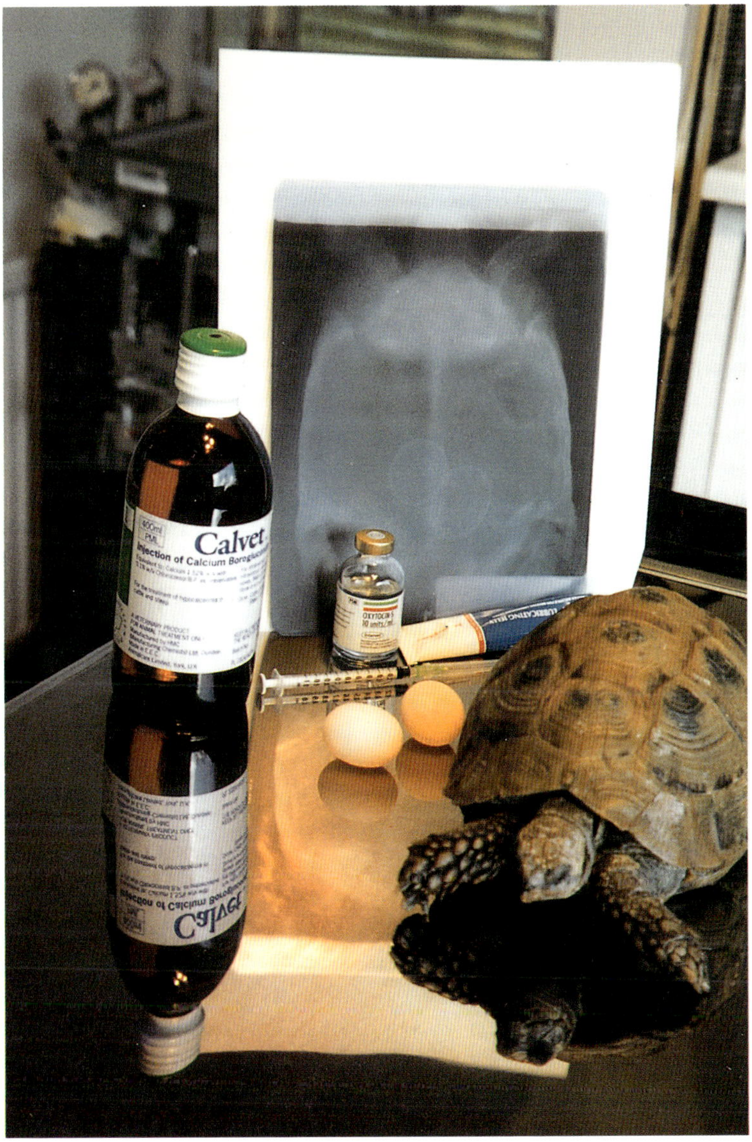


**Plate 36** The requirements for medical management of egg retention are easily met by most practices. This tortoise was never hibernated and regularly laid eggs each November. By late March she had become unusually anorexic. Occasional puffing, rocking and straining observed by the owner had been put down to constipation. Radiography revealed two large coelomic eggs. The treatment given consisted of cloacal lubrication and a calcium injection followed by an oxytocin injection 12 hours later. Both eggs were passed within four hours of the oxytocin injection and normal behaviour and appetite resumed within ten days of treatment.

### *Environmental considerations*

**Assess the environment for possible problems and correct them**

- Temperature
- Photoperiod
- Diet
- Availability of fresh water
- Humidity
- Human interventions
- Housing with aggressive males

### *Medical treatment*

Oxytocin has been used with great success in tortoises. It must only be used where no obstruction to the passage of eggs through the pelvic canal (e.g. a cloacal calculus) is present, or oviductal rupture with resultant egg peritonitis and death may occur.

**Advice concerning medical management of egg retention**

- Cloacal lubrication with a suitable obstetric lubricant is advised before starting treatment. I try and do this 24 hours before giving any medication.
- Calcium gluconate should be given at 0.5–1.0 mg/kg body weight to complement any oxytocin given later. Most authors advise this solution precede the oxytocin solution by several hours. I try and give it in the evening and then give oxytocin the following day.
- 1–5 IU of oxytocin/kg bodyweight have been advised intramuscularly by a variety of authors. Avoid the rapid use of high doses as oviductal spasm and secondary rupture are more likely. (I find 1 IU/kg is often adequate.)
- 50% of this dose may be repeated four hours later if egg expulsion has not yet occurred.
- Advice on continued medical management varies. Most authors seem to advise that oxytocin be repeated cautiously and suggest calcium gluconate therapy on its own instead.

### *Surgical treatment*

Where egg retention as a result of abnormally large eggs, abnormally shaped eggs or failure of medical management has occurred, coeliotomy as described in the section on 'Surgical techniques and shell repairs' can be performed. Medical management should be attempted cautiously if radiography shows the passage of eggs to be potentially impossible.

Finally, if presented with a single large egg in the pelvic inlet that appears too large to be passed despite lubrication and hormonal treatments and perhaps the client is unable to afford a coeliotomy, or the facilities are not available, then it may be possible to perform careful cloacal puncture of the offending egg. Its contents, often grossly infected, may be carefully aspirated. The cloaca should then be flushed with antibiotics or disinfectant solutions (e.g. Pevidine: C-Vet). Expulsion of debris may be assisted by the use of calcium, oxytocin and lubrication as described above.

# THE NATURAL ENVIRONMENT AND HUSBANDRY OF CHELONIA

It must be remembered that the client may often know more about the needs of an unusual pet than the veterinarian and this is a useful source of information. If the client is unable to explain where the animal can normally be found, what it is like in this place, and what must be provided when kept in different environments, then it may follow that the animal is not being supplied with the husbandry necessary for its survival.

The following Chelonia are considered in this section:

Red-eared terrapin/slider/turtle (*Pseudemys scripta elegans*)
European pond terrapin/turtle (*Emrys orbicularis*)
American box turtle/tortoise (*Terrapene* spp.)
Asiatic box turtle
African hingeback tortoise (*Kinyxis* spp.)
Leopard tortoise (*Geochelone pardalis*)
Redfoot tortoise (*Geochelone carbonaria*)
Mediterranean species of tortoise (*Testudo* spp.).

## RED-EARED TERRAPIN/SLIDER/TURTLE (*Pseudemys scripta elegans*)

These animals are currently quite popular with the general public. Whilst they start as small easily managed animals (of just a few centimetres) they soon grow to a large size (up to 30 cm). They require special accommodation such as a tank with water filtration, lighting and heating. There are currently a surplus of such animals requiring rehoming and a shortage of willing new homes.

Current trade in these animals involves the exportation of 3–4 million animals a year from intensive farms in southern USA; a very large number of which will die within 3–6 months. There are strong moves to try and restrict and control this trade, and educate the public as to the unsuitability of these animals as pets.

**Diet**

- Terrapins are omnivorous and thrive on both animal and plant material in suitable combinations. This is discussed in the 'Nutrition' section. Mineral and vitamin deficiencies are common in these animals and a regular supplement is advised.
- Diets that centre around animal protein tend to have a high phosphorus level in relation to calcium and this may well result in abnormal shell and bone growth. Supplementation with some accessible form of calcium such as Nutrobal will counteract this, as will offering cuttlefish bone to be gnawed.

**Juvenile accommodation**

- Small terrapins less than 10 cm are best kept in a heated aquarium. The size of this aquarium will relate to the size and number of terrapins, but a surface area allowance of about 900 square centimetres surface area per 10 cm terrapin is suitable.
- The water depth should allow the terrapin to submerge and swim about. Small terrapins less than 5 cm long should not be kept in water deeper than 5 cm.
- The terrarium should have an area where rocks, logs or land is provided. This should also have a small basking area.
- The water temperature should be about 23–30°C during the day and this should fall to about 16°C at night. A thermostatically controlled heater is helpful here.

**Adult accommodation**

- Adult terrapins with a shell length greater than 10 cm can be kept outdoors in a garden pond, particularly in the warm southern counties. The pond should have a minimum surface area of 1 metre square per terrapin.
- The sides should slope to assist in exiting the water.
- A damp and shady covering is preferred with a brighter area for basking in the sun.
- As turtles are excellent climbers a fence about 30 cm high with a buried base is essential. Some animals constantly climb such a fence and these will often stop if a solid wall is used. The run should be dog and fox proof.
- Terrapins should be acclimatized for a period of three weeks or more before introduction to a cold water outdoor environment. This is best done in spring or summer.
- A large indoor vivarium is also suitable as described above in 'Juvenile accommodation', the area allowances will need to be increased.

**Water quality**

- Water quality has a great effect on the health of these animals.
- The incidence of bacterial and parasitic diseases will increase rapidly when this is not attended to as it becomes heavily contaminated with excreta.
- A motorized filtration system is of help in maintaining hygiene.
- Regular water changes should be arranged at least once a week. A vivarium should be cleaned and scrubbed at the same time.

**Hibernation**

- Small animals kept in tanks as described above do not generally require hibernation.
- Outdoor animals will often do very well without hibernation. If the pond is likely to freeze over the terrapin can be put into a resting state at about 5°C in a moist but well-ventilated box or enclosure.

## EUROPEAN POND TERRAPIN/TURTLE (*Emrys orbicularis*)

This terrapin comes from central and southern Europe, North-west Africa and Western Asia. It is a very hardy species and is dark green or black with small yellow spots on its head. It requires similar conditions to those described for the red-eared terrapin but copes better at cooler temperatures.

## AMERICAN BOX TURTLES/TORTOISES (*Terrapene* spp).

These are semi-aquatic tortoises. They are easily identified by their unusually mobile plastral hinges which, in non-obese animals, enable them to withdraw tightly behind a protective 'drawbridge' so that not even limbs are exposed.

There are various species of box turtles but the type most commonly seen in this country if *Terrapene carolina triungus* (the three-toed box turtle).

Sexing of these animals is not easy, but males tend to have a red iris and females a yellow or brown iris.

**Captive environment**

- This must be kept very humid.
- They should be maintained in a warm environment at about 18–27°C.
- If kept outside any enclosure must be escape-proof, as these animals enjoy burrowing and climbing.
- Box turtles should be kept indoors in ideal conditions upon their first entry to the UK.
- They should not be hibernated during their first year in this country.
- They may be acclimatized to an outdoor terrarium gradually by starting in spring with protection at night and during cold weather. Such animals will have a long hibernation if kept outside over the winter.
- If animals are kept indoors then a Philips 'Tru-Lite' fluorescent strip light is advised to compensate for lack of natural daylight.
- Soil or suitable substrate should be provided as these animals enjoy burrowing. This should be changed regularly to avoid excessive bacterial contamination. It should also be escape-proof.

**Hibernation**

- A high humidity is required.
- A maximum of three months is advised.
- Box turtles are very vulnerable to low temperatures and the hibernation site should be well protected.
- Animals kept indoors in a suitable environment do not require hibernation.
- Newly imported animals should not be hibernated in their first year.

**Diet**

- Young *Terrapene* spp. are particularly carnivorous but as they mature the tendency is for a higher proportion of vegetable matter to be consumed. More mature animals will also require fruit and vegetables.
- A vitamin supplement such as Nutrobal: Vetark Professional, Vionate: Sherleys or ACE-High: Vetark Professional is advised daily.
- A small amount of meat, fish or low fat dog food may be offered occasionally. The fat content of some cat and dog foods is particularly high and these should be avoided.

## Handling

The application of pressure to the posterior plastron generally allows the anterior plastron to be opened. The limbs and head can usually be drawn out one after another to allow examination. A rubber eraser can assist in preventing the animal's retreat but handling can be quite difficult. Observation from a distance may be unavoidable.

### Health considerations

Most of the infectious health problems discussed with Mediterranean tortoises also occur with box tortoises and treatment is very similar. Recently imported animals should be kept separate from other Chelonia and screened for problems such as:

- *Hexamita* infection
- helminth infection
- ectoparasites

before any contact with existing stock is allowed.

### Environmental influences and anorexia

Box turtles are particularly sensitive to environmental conditions. A recently imported box turtle kept in a garden will often be presented as anorexic, but if returned to the correct temperature and humidity will resume eating.

### Heat, light and humidity

Box turtles do not tolerate excessive radiant heat or constant exposure to bright light. Such conditions appear to encourage ear, eye and respiratory infections. Any animal under treatment for such a condition should have its environment assessed.

## ASIATIC BOX TURTLES

There are various species and they differ from American box turtles in that they prefer a higher ambient temperature range 27–30°C. Asiatic box turtles do not cope outside and require a vivarium. They should not be hibernated.

## AFRICAN HINGEBACK TORTOISE (*Kinyxis* spp.)

All hingeback tortoises are characterized by a distinct single hinge located about three quarters of the way along the back of the tortoise. It is the carapace and ***not*** the plastron that is hinged. This makes the distinction between hingeback and box tortoises straightforward.

**Environment**

- All species require a constantly warm environment at about 27–28°C.
- All hingeback tortoises must be provided with constant access to water (a bathing and a drinking area).
- Most hingebacks require a high level of humidity. Avoid bright lights or drying heat sources (occasional spraying with a mist from a plant spray and the inclusion of ample damp substrates).
- As hingebacks will spend the majority of time in a relatively permanent vivarium, it should be well planned, illuminated with 'Tru-lite' or similar full spectrum fluorescent tubes and be relatively spacious with ample leafy cover.

**Diet**

- African hingebacks are omnivorous and insectivorous. Their preferred diet is included in the 'Nutrition' section.
- A small amount of low fat dog food can be offered occasionally (about once a week).
- A calcium-rich supplement such as Nutrobal: Vetark Professional is advised.

**Health considerations**

- As was described with box turtles. Recently imported animals should always be screened for parasitic and infectious diseases prior to mixing with existing stock. Nematodes, protozoan infections and external parasites are all common and should be eliminated.
- If a sub-optimal environment is provided anorexia will result.
- A dry environment will precipitate eye, ear, and respiratory infections.

### Hibernation

These animals should *never* be hibernated. A moist vivarium is essential throughout the winter.

## LEOPARD TORTOISE (*Geochelone pardalis*)

The leopard tortoise is a large African species and specimens of 700 mm long and 40 kg have been recorded. They require extensive accommodation and a large volume of suitable foods.

### Accommodation

| | |
|---|---|
| **Juveniles** | • Small specimens cope well in a large well-lit and heated vivarium.<br>• Background temperatures are about 24°C day and 16°C at night.<br>• A separate 'hot-spot' in the region of 30°C should be provided by the use of a 100 W spot lamp or 100 W ceramic infra-red heater.<br>• 'Tru-lite' full spectrum fluorescent tubes (48/40 W) are excellent.<br>• 'Sun-Glo' or 'Northlight/Actinic' U/V are also of use.<br>• Adequate lighting is essential. |
| **Adolescents/ adults** | • With the rapid growth of this species a large indoor pen is soon required (2.5 m × 2.5 m) with suitable heating and lighting suspended above it. |
| **Humidity** | • This must not be excessively high.<br>• A warm moderately dry environment minimizes respiratory problems.<br>• Ventilation should be maintained and pens should be open-topped. |
| **Outdoor environment** | • These animals enjoy grazing outside during good weather. |

| Diet |
|---|
| • Leopard tortoises eat a wide range of fruit and as wide a variety of choice as possible should be offered.<br>• These animals enjoy access to grasses, cabbages, and other green leaf vegetables in reasonable quantities. These animals benefit from a high fibre diet. |

### Disease predisposition

It is essential to quarantine animals before their introduction into existing colonies. Diseases such as *Hexamita* spp. infestation, helminthiasis and ectoparasites are not uncommon.

These animals suffer most of the conditions included in this manual and treatment will be similar to that for Mediterranean species.

## REDFOOT TORTOISES (*Geochelone carbonaria*)

Most adults measure about 300–350 mm and weigh about 5–6 kg. These tropical tortoises are found from Argentina to Panama and have colonized many Caribbean islands and are the most common south American tortoise. They are recognized by the bright red scales on their legs giving them their name.

| | |
|---|---|
| **Accommodation** | • These animals require a reasonable level of humidity and benefit from a 'tropical greenhouse environment'. They do not enjoy bright lights and enjoy low light intensity within a vivarium maintained at a constant 28–29°C.<br>• These animals should be kept indoors but will enjoy occasional periods outside provided that they have access to shade and the weather is suitable. |
| **Diet** | • They are herbivorous tortoises that enjoy a high fruit component to the diet. Constant access to drinking water is essential. |

## MEDITERRANEAN SPECIES OF TORTOISE (*Testudo* spp.)

| | *Testudo hermanni* | *Testudo (graeca) ibera* |
|---|---|---|
| **Importation controls** | Yes | Yes |
| **UK prevalence** | Relatively common | Relatively common |
| **Specific features of species** | Horny tip to tail (Tubercle) | Tubercle on medial thigh |
| **Usual adult size**<br>**Male**<br>**Female** | Medium<br>120–165 mm<br>130–190 mm | Medium<br>~180 mm<br>~210 mm |
| **Sexing advice** | Males are usually smaller, have a longer tail and a concave plastron. | Males are usually smaller, have a longer tail and a concave plastron. |
| **Countries of origin** | Southern Europe (Mediterranean) Spain, France, Italy, Yugoslavia, Greece, Turkey. | Eastern Europe and the Middle East Turkey, Bulgaria, Romania, Iran, Jordan, Georgia. |
| **Natural environment** | Mediterranean evergreen and oak forests, also herbaceous scrub where forests have declined. | Mediterranean evergreen and oak forests, also herbaceous scrub where forests have declined. |
| **Suitable captive environment (summer)** | Will cope outdoors in well drained herbaceous areas that are protected and enclosed. Sheltered sleeping quarters should be provided. | (Like *T. hermanni*) These animals are quite robust and cope reasonably well with significant climatic variations. |
| **Natural diet in the wild** | Succulent and herbaceous plants. The diet is high in fibre. It tends to be moist in spring and autumn but very dry in summer. | Succulent and herbaceous plants. The diet is high in fibre. It tends to be moist in spring and autumn but very dry in summer. |
| **Hibernation** | Tends to be November to April in a suitably prepared area. Never expose these animals to sub-zero temperatures. | Tends to be November to April in a suitably prepared area. Never expose these animals to sub-zero temperatures. |

| | *Testudo graeca graeca* | *Testudo marginata* |
|---|---|---|
| **Importation controls** | Yes | Yes |
| **UK prevalence** | Becoming quite rare | Relatively common |
| **Specific features of species** | Tubercle on medial thigh | Flared posterior marginal scutes |
| **Usual adult size** | Small | Large |
| **Male** | ~130 mm | 250–295 mm |
| **Female** | ~160 mm | 240–300 mm |
| **Sexing advice** | Males are usually smaller, have a longer tail and a concave plastron. | Females tend to be broader and heavier. |
| **Countries of origin** | Morocco, Algeria, and southern Spain | Greece |
| **Natural environment** | Environment seasonally varies between 60° and 90°F. Animals may aestivate underground in the heat of summer. | Mediterranean evergreen and oak forests, also herbaceous scrub where forests have declined. |
| **Suitable captive environment (summer)** | This tortoise does not mix well with other species. It is particularly sensitive to climatic variations. It does better with high humidity. | (Like *T. hermanni*) These animals are quite robust and cope reasonably well with significant climatic variations. |
| **Natural diet in the wild** | Similar to the others but consumes a higher proportion of flowers. | Succulent and herbaceous plants. The diet is high in fibre. It tends to be moist in spring and autumn but very dry in summer. |
| **Hibernation** | Keep hibernation short, this species does not cope so well in captivity. Heat and light can be supplemented at the start and end of hibernation in order to restrict its duration. | Tends to be November to April in a suitably prepared area. Never expose these animals to sub-zero temperatures. |

# EUTHANASIA

This is seldom requested and there is very little information available on the subject. Indeed the assessment of death in an animal capable of hibernation is not easy.

| Criteria for diagnosing death include |
| --- |
| • Absence of heartbeat using ECG, pulse oximetry |
| • Absence of respiration |
| • Absence of response to stimulus, e.g. corneal reflexes |
| • Absence of response to warming if chilled |
| • Rigor mortis |
| • Grey/cyanotic mucous membrane colour |
| • Postmortem tissue necrosis |
| • Sunken, deflated eyes |

Obviously there are times where euthanasia, as an emergency or out of humanity, is required. The following are suggestions and their vagueness relates to the limited amount of published material concerning this subject. I tend to use intravenous pentobarbitone. Premedication with ketamine facilitates intravenous injections in box turtles and active animals and makes the whole situation far less distressing for any client present.

## LETHAL INJECTION

| | Comments |
| --- | --- |
| **Pentobarbitone** | This can be used in conjunction with other methods. I tend to give a premedication dose of ketamine i.m. and follow this with an intravenous injection of 200 mg/kg pentobarbitone solution. This has proven consistently effective and is currently my method of choice. |
| **Chloroform** | ? Irritant/painful by injection, used in very old texts.<br>? Intracardiac–intracoelomic–intravenous. |

## SATURATION OF AIRSPACE

This can be achieved by placing the tortoise in a closed contained containing a small amount of halothane, chloroform or ether. Sometimes only a short exposure is required but the time taken will vary. It must be remembered that reptiles are capable of hibernation and survival at very low metabolic rates. They may survive by anaerobic respiration for some considerable time. This is particularly true of aquatic species. ***I do not advise this method unless no other option is available. Care should be taken to minimize human health hazards from toxicity and explosion.***

## FREEZING AND DECAPITATION

Although this method is advised by some older texts, it is not particularly humane. Chilled animals may still perceive pain. Decapitated animals may retain brain function to varying degrees for some considerable time unless pithed immediately. ***This method is not advised unless no other option is available.***

# THERAPEUTICS

The following information has been collected from various sources. I have tried to identify these wherever possible.

- The weight of a tortoise shell does not need to be subtracted when calculating drug doses (Lawrence 1984).
- All doses are safe and accurate to the best of my knowledge at the time of writing, provided hydration, maintenance temperature, duration of treatment, and route of administration are also considered.
- The drugs and doses advised are not licensed for use in the tortoise and no responsibility is taken by the author should any legal matter arise from using them. It is advised that clients are asked to sign a consent form for the use of an unlicensed product, such as that produced by the Veterinary Defence Society, before any animal is treated to cover against any subsequent litigation.
- An alternative system of drug dose calculation is given in the *BSAVA Manual of Reptiles*. As the method involves a scaling of the dose that relates to the volume of the animal it is likely to be more accurate than the empirical doses given in this text should it enter common use.
- Treatment of Gram-negative infections may predispose to a massive endotoxin release during initial treatments. This must be closely monitored.

## TEMPERATURE

It should be noted that most medications are best given with the patient being maintained at a constant temperature. This is usually in the region of its ***preferred optimum temperature***. As the tortoise is an ectotherm, drug activity and metabolism are dramatically affected by temperature. The usual maintenance temperature is 24–30°C but where specific information is available I have included it. Most problems occur with drugs such as anaesthetics and the nephrotoxic aminoglycosides. Small variations in temperatures seriously affect the half-life of any drug given.

It is essential to keep these animals reasonably warm during periods of hospitalization.

## HYDRATION

Fluid supplementation is recommended to decrease the toxic effects of certain groups of drugs, particularly anaesthetic agents, neuromuscular blocking agents and the aminoglycoside antibiotics. This supplementation is usually via oral administration/stomach tubing. It is wise to address this problem whenever dehydration as a result of debility is considered to be present. Volumes comparable to those given in the table for force feeding may be used. The type of fluid used varies. If diuresis is desired, hypotonic solutions such as water are used. If rehydration is desired, one may want to use a solution such as Hartmann's or diluted Liquid Lectade.

## DRUG INTERACTIONS/TOXICITIES

The following drugs should be used with caution. More complete explanations regarding their use are given elsewhere in the text and in the 'Drugs and dosages' section that follows.

| |
|---|
| Ketamine (debility) |
| Succinylcholine chloride (interactions) |
| Aminoglycosides (interactions) |
| Frusemide (interactions) |
| Ivermectin (toxic) |
| Piperazine (toxic) |
| Oxytetraclines (may precipitate SGS) |

### The use of chloramphenicol

Whilst included in many sensitivity tests performed by commercial laboratories, this drug has a reserve status for treatment of human *Salmonella* infections. It is usually possible to find a more suitable drug with a bacteriocidal, as opposed to a bacteriostatic, action.

### Prophylactic use of ketoconazole

Some authors (e.g. Page & Mautino 1990) currently favour the concurrent use of ketoconazole at a dose rate of 30 mg/kg orally daily for 2–4 weeks when treating bacterial infections with potent antibiotics that may seriously affect bacterial flora. Prophylactic therapies should always be looked into carefully as they may encourage resistance and superinfection with yet further unpleasant organisms. However, their use may well be justified in some situations.

### Treatment of *Salmonella* and *Campylobacter* infections

In view of the zoonotic potential of these infections animals from whom these organisms have been isolated should always be treated to eliminate even a symptomless infection. The prevalence of both organisms is particularly low and the following drug regime has been effective: ampicillin 75 mg/tortoise and chloramphenicol 250 mg/tortoise for ten days (Zwart 1987). The possibility of carriers requires consideration. Animals suspected of carrying these diseases do not make suitable pets for children, the elderly, or immunosuppressed individuals even after they are treated. Wherever possible the antibiotic is best chosen after performing a culture and sensitivity test of the pathogen.

### Choice of antibiotic

Bacteriocidal antibiotics should be used in preference to bacteriostatic antibiotics wherever possible. This is especially true where underlying immunosuppression is suspected.

When changing an ineffective antibiotic one should take care if following a bacteriostatic antibiotic with a bacteriocidal as there may only be a limited number of dividing bacteria on which the bacteriocidal may act.

### Prophylactic probiotic solutions

These may be used if SGS or fungal superinfection is anticipated. See 'Mycotic enteritis' in the section on 'Fungal infections' and 'Sterile gut syndrome' in the section on 'Bacterial infections'.

# DRUGS AND DOSAGES

## PREMEDICANT/ANAESTHETIC/RESTRAINING DRUGS

**Acepromazine** (Various preparations)

| | |
|---|---|
| Route: | Intramuscular injection. |
| Dose: | 0.1–0.5 mg/kg. |
| Information: | Dose given is for 'reptile' and I have no experience of this with Chelonia. It may be parallel to mammalian sedation. |
| Source: | Frye (1991). |

**Alphaxalone/Alphadolone** (Saffan: Mallinckrodt)

| | |
|---|---|
| Route: | I.V. if possible.<br>I.M. but not as reliable (prolonged induction time). |
| Dose: | 9 mg/kg i.v.<br>12–18 mg/kg i.m. (15 mg/kg average). |
| Information: | Predictable results that allow intubation and maintenance with gaseous anaesthesia. I.V. anaesthesia lasts in the region of ten or more minutes and allows simple procedures to be performed. Intramuscular route tends to result in delayed onset and may fail to fully reach surgical anaesthesia. It is possible to cautiously supplement the i.m. dose with a very much reduced i.v. dose, to effect, as this is much easier in the sedated/partially anaesthetized animal. Intubation, intermittent positive pressure ventilation (IPPV), and close observation/monitoring are advised to prevent overdose. |
| Source: | Cooper & Beynon (1991); Lawrence & Jackson (1983b). |

**Atropine sulphate** (Various preparations)

Route: Subcutaneous injection.

Dose: 0.01–0.04 mg/kg.

Information: Dose given is for 'reptile', nothing specific given for Chelonia. It may act as one would expect in the mammal.

Source: Frye (1991).

**Ketamine** (Various, e.g. Vatalar: Parke-Davis)

Route: Intramuscular into thoracic limb.

Dose: Suggested doses vary between 20–100 mg/kg.

Information: Low doses have been used to facilitate gaseous anaesthesia via intubation or an induction chamber, however there are many risks and considerations acknowledged with this agent:

(1) Variable plane of anaesthesia/analgesia. Some animals appear to continue movements etc. throughout the period of activity, others go unreasonably inactive. Sometimes the recovery period can be measured in days. Dose is significant.

(2) Do not use if dehydrated, debilitated, or if hepatic or renal disease may be present, as the result may be unpredictable and stress may seriously complicate any underlying condition.

(3) Personality changes have been reported in some reptiles.

(4) Apparently it should be given into the thoracic limb as renal portal flow results in excessive drug levels reaching viscera.

Source: Cooper & Beynon (1991); Frye (1991); Rübel (1991); Page & Mautino (1990).

**Lignocaine** (Various preparations)

Route: Local infiltration.

Dose: To effect, minimum effective dose.

Information: May be used in combination with ketamine, alphaxalone/alphadolone, succinylcholine chloride, etc. No toxic side effects noted.

Source: Frye (1991); Holt *et al.* (1979).

**Propofol** (Rapinovet: Mallinckrodt)

Route: I.V. injection only (slow injection).

Dose: 1–1.4 ml/kg.

Information: A short-acting knock-down drug usually followed by intubation and gaseous anaesthesia. Prolonged apnoea can be seen in chelonians treated with this drug, particularly if the propofol is given rapidly. A slow dose to effect policy will reduce this problem.

Source: Cooper & Beynon (1991).

**Succinylcholine chloride** (Human preparations)

Route: Intramuscular injection into thoracic limb.

Dose: 0.25–1.5 mg/kg

Information:

(1) Do not use in combination with aminoglycoside antibiotics or other nephrotoxic drugs.

(2) No analgesia. Perhaps combine with local anaesthetic or use for immobilization/examination only. The drug may cause distress that we are unable to assess.

(3) Ventilation is likely to be required and this may involve intubation or artificial limb movements.

***Use with care as it has no analgesia; it may distress the animal. Its use may not be ethical.***

Source: Page & Mautino (1990).

## GASEOUS/VOLATILE ANAESTHETICS

**Halothane** (Various preparations)

Route: Inhalation.

Dose: In region of 0.5–3% or as required.

Information: Intubate and use $O_2 : NO_2$ as vector to transport in 1:2 ratio. Induce with an injectable anaesthetic. IPPV may be required.

Source: Cooper & Beynon (1991).

**Isoflurane** (Various preparations)

Route: Inhalation.

Dose: In the region of 0.5–1.5%.

Information: Where available, the excellent control of anaesthetic depth and recovery make this the anaesthetic of choice for most exotics including reptiles. As it is not particularly metabolized by the patient it is of great use in debilitated animals such as those in renal or hepatic failure. IPPV may be required.

Source: D. Williams and R. Hummond RVC (1994), personal communication.

**Methoxyflurane** (Various preparations)

Route: Inhalation.

Dose: Not specified, 'low concentrations' referred to.

Information: Intube and use $O_2 : NO_2$ as vector to transport in 1:2 ratio. Induce with an injectable anaesthetic. IPPV may be required.

Source: Cooper & Beynon (1991).

**Nitrous oxide**

Route: Inhalation.

Dose: Two parts $NO_2$ to one part $O_2$ as maintenance gas composition.

Information: Decreases the amount of volatile anaesthetic required for maintenance.

Source: Cooper & Beynon (1991).

## AGENTS USED FOR EUTHANASIA

**Chloroform/halothane/ether** (Various preparations)

Route: Intracoelomic injection or inhalation with excess liquid in a sealed box. Death may be prolonged due to anaerobic respiration.

Information: Ensure operator safety (provide ventilation). Monitor this procedure carefully.

Source: Older texts.

**Pentobarbitone** (Lethobarb: Solvay Duphar; Euthesate: Willows Francis, etc.)

| | |
|---|---|
| Route: | Intravenous injection/intracardiac injection. |
| Dose: | To excess. 1 ml/kg of the above solutions (200 mg/ml). |
| Information: | Results may not prove consistent or reliable as death may be unduly prolonged if a rapid blood level is not achieved. I tend to immobilize animals such as terrapins or box turtles with ketamine at a high dose. This facilitates subsequent intravenous pentobarbitone injection. |
| Source: | Accepted use of product. |

## VITAMIN PREPARATIONS BY INJECTION

**Vitamin A** (Retinol)

| | |
|---|---|
| Route: | Intramuscular injection. |
| Dose: | 1000–5000 IU weekly in known deficiency.<br>10 000–20 000 IU as a single dose. |
| Information: | Oral supplementation should be undertaken as a constant low level input is desirable and toxicity is rapidly achieved with repeated injections. Fat soluble. Little of this vitamin is stored. Toxicity manifests as skin sloughing. |
| Source: | Cooper & Beynon (1991); Highfield (1990); Page & Mautino (1990); Lawton (1987); Zwart (1987). |

**Vitamin B** (complex)

| | |
|---|---|
| Route: | Intramuscular or subcuticular injection. |
| Dose: | 0.25–0.5 mg/kg. |
| Information: | Frequency and indications not established. |
| Source: | Frye (1991). |

**Vitamin $B_1$** (Thiamine)

| | |
|---|---|
| Route: | Oral |
| Dose: | 25 mg/kg. |
| Information: | Frequency not established. May be of use in anaemia. |
| Source: | Cooper & Beynon (1991). |

**Vitamin $B_{12}$** (Cyanocolbamin)

Route: Intramuscular or subcuticular.

Dose: Vaguely described as 2000–10 000 mg/tortoise or 0.5 mg/kg.

Information: Frequency not described, may be used as appetite stimulant but not yet proven to be effective.

Source: Cooper & Beynon (1991); Frye (1991); Page & Mautino (1990).

**Vitamin C** (Ascorbic acid)

Route: Intramuscular injection.

Dosage: 10–20 mg/kg (daily when required).

Information: This has been suggested to be of benefit during bacterial infections to complement the use of antibiotics. No adverse reactions are described. A true vitamin C deficiency has not yet been documented to the best of my knowledge.

Source: Frye (1991); Highfield (1990); Page & Mautino (1990).

**Vitamin $D_3$**

Route: Intramuscular injection.

Dose: 1500–1650 IU/kg as a single dose.

Information: Repeat doses may result in toxicity. Address any underlying cause, e.g. unsuitable nutrition, exposure to natural daylight. Supplement further orally if required.

Source: Highfield (1990); Page & Mautino (1990); Zwart (1987).

**Vitamin ADE** (Combination) (Jectadine: Beecham Animal Health)

Route: Intramuscular.

Dose: 0.2 ml/kg as a single dose.

Information: Repeat doses may result in toxicity. Address any underlying cause. Supplement further orally if required.

Source: Cooper *et al.* (1990).

## VARIOUS NON-ANTIBIOTIC DRUGS

**Apomorphine**

| | |
|---|---|
| Route: | Intramuscular injection. |
| Dose: | 0.35 mg/kg single dose. |
| Information: | Initial marked drowsiness followed by increased appetite was recorded. No emetic effects noted. Safety margins not established especially in debility. |
| Source: | Zwart & Buitelaar (1980). |

**Dexamethasone** (Azium: Schering Plough; Dexadreson: Intervet)

| | |
|---|---|
| Route: | Intravenous or intramuscular injection. |
| Dose: | 0.125–0.6 mg/kg. |
| Informaion: | Frequency as needed. Indications have not been established. Should not be used unless any underlying infections are receiving appropriate therapy. Should not be used where immunosuppression is likely to exacerbate the condition. |
| Source: | Frye (1991). |

**Frusemide** (Lasix: Hoechst)

| | |
|---|---|
| Route: | Intravenous or intramuscular injection. |
| Dose: | 5 mg/kg. |
| Information: | Frequency as required. Contraindicated with aminoglycoside therapy. |
| Source: | Cooper & Beynon (1991); Frye (1991). |

**Methionine** (Evans)

| | |
|---|---|
| Route: | Orally. |
| Dose: | 200–250 mg/tortoise every 48 hours. |
| Information: | To aid the treatment of hepatitis/steatitis. |
| Source: | Cooper & Beynon (1991); Highfield (1990). |

**Nandrolone phenylproprionate** (Nandrolin injection: Intervet)

| | |
|---|---|
| Route: | Intramuscular injection. |
| Dose: | 0.5 mg/tortoise. |
| Information: | Weekly, for as long as several months if appropriate. Indications include hepatitis, fatty liver, renal disease and non-specific debility. |
| Source: | Cooper & Beynon (1991). |

**L-thyroxine sodium** (Soloxine: Daniels Pharmaceuticals)

| | |
|---|---|
| Route: | Orally. |
| Dose: | 0.2 mg/tortoise every 48 hours. |
| Information: | May be of use in any fatty liver/iodine linked problem. |
| Source: | Beynon *et al.* (1992); Cooper & Beynon (1991). |

## REPRODUCTIVE THERAPY

**Calcium borogluconate** (Various preparations)

| | |
|---|---|
| Route: | Intramuscular injection. |
| Dose: | 1 ml/kg of a 1% solution and 0.5 ml/kg of a 10% solution have both been advised. The dose is normally repeated daily over several days if needed. |
| Information: | Should precede oxytocin by 24 hours if inducing oviposition. It is repeated daily. In cases of nutritional osteodystrophic treatment it is more important to address nutrition and environment as a whole than to provide excessive calcium by injection. |
| Source: | Beynon (1992); Cooper & Beynon (1991); Highfield (1990); Muller *et al.* (1989). |

**Oxytocin** (Oxytocin-S: Intervet; various others)

| | |
|---|---|
| Route: | Intramuscular injection. |
| Dose: | 1 IU, 1.5–10 IU, 2–10 IU and $< 3$ IU per kg have all been advised. I find 1 IU/kg is usually adequate. |
| Information: | In conjunction with concurrent daily calcium borogluconate. Can be repeated but frequency is not well defined. Every three days may be suitable. Do not use if obstruction to passage of eggs has not been corrected.<br>Care should be taken as oviductal spasm and rupture can occur at higher dosages.<br>It is wise to consider environmental causes for delayed oviposition. |
| Source: | Beynon (1992); Cooper & Beynon (1991); Highfield (1990); Muller *et al.* (1989). |

## ANTHELMINTIC PREPARATIONS

**Albendazole** (Valbenzen: SmithKline Beecham)

| | |
|---|---|
| Route: | Orally (via stomach tube). |
| Dose: | 50–75 mg/kg. |
| Information: | Minimum dose of 1 ml/tortoise. |
| Source: | Cooper & Beynon (1991). |

**Fenbendazole** (Panacur: Hoechst)

| | |
|---|---|
| Route: | Orally (via stomach tube). |
| Dose: | 50–100 mg/kg repeated at two weeks. |
| Information: | May not eliminate whole worm burden even with two doses, but safe and reasonably effective. Usually a minimum dose of 1 ml/tortoise is given. |
| Source: | Cooper & Beynon (1991); Frye (1991); Page & Mautino (1990). |

**Ivermectin** (Ivomec: MSD Agvet)

| | |
|---|---|
| Route: | Not suitable. |
| Dose: | Not suitable. |
| Information: | Has proved fatal. |
| Source: | Cooper & Beynon (1991); Teare & Bush (1983). |

**Oxfendazole** (Systemex: Mallinckrodt)

| | |
|---|---|
| Route: | Orally (via stomach tube). |
| Dose: | 65 mg/kg as a single dose. This is about 3 ml/kg of a 2.256% solution. |
| Information: | Usually a minimum dose of 1 ml/tortoise is given. The wormer of choice, as low side effects and high efficacy against all helminths at a single dose. |
| Source: | Cooper & Beynon (1991); Highfield (1990); Lawton (1987). |

**Piperazine** (Various preparations)

| | |
|---|---|
| Route: | Not suitable. |
| Dose: | Not suitable. |
| Information: | Toxic and ineffective. |
| Source: | Highfield (1990). |

## ANTIFUNGAL PREPARATIONS

**Ketoconazole** (Nizoral: Janssen)

| | |
|---|---|
| Route: | Orally. |
| Dose: | 15–30 mg/kg daily. |
| Information: | Used simultaneously with any broad-spectrum antibiotic therapy to prevent possible fungal overgrowth/superinfection. Used as an antifungal preparation in its own right. No toxic effects noted at this dose. |
| Source: | Page & Mautino (1990); Page *et al.* (1988). |

**Malachite green**

| | |
|---|---|
| Route: | External/topical. |
| Dose: | Paint lesions with a 2 mg/litre solution. |
| Information: | Ulcerative shell disease of fungal origin. |
| Source: | Highfield (1990); Zwart (1987). |

**Nystatin** (Panalog: Ciba Animal Health)

| | |
|---|---|
| Route: | Orally (topical use is mentioned elsewhere in this text). |
| Dose: | 0.2–0.3 ml daily for 10–15 days. |
| Information: | The steroidal component may not be advantageous in animals where immunosuppression is suspected. Its use is limited to gastrointestinal infections as it is very poorly absorbed. |
| Source: | Zwart & Buitelaar (1980). |

**Povidone-iodine** (Pevidine: C-Vet; Betadine: Seton).

| | |
|---|---|
| Route: | External/topical only. |
| Dose: | As required, undiluted or diluted 50 : 50 with water. |
| Information: | Excellent routine disinfectant, surgical scrub, and of great use in necrotic stomatitis/ulcerative shell disease. |
| Source: | Acceptable use of product. |

## ANTIVIRAL PREPARATIONS

**Acyclovir** (Zovirax 5% w/w: Wellcome)

| | |
|---|---|
| Route: | Topical. |
| Dose: | According to lesion size, daily. |
| Information: | Good results were achieved in cases of necrotic-stomatitis assumed to have an underlying herpes virus aetiology. |
| Source: | Frye (1991); Cooper *et al.* (1988). |

## ECTOPARASITIDES

**Amitraz** (Aludex: Hoechst)

| | |
|---|---|
| Route: | Local application. |
| Dose: | Dilute 2 ml/litre and wash with emulsion. |
| Source: | Petney & Knight (1988). |

## ANTIPROTOZOAN DRUGS

**Dimetronidazole** (Emytryl: Rhône Mérieux)

| | |
|---|---|
| Route: | Orally. |
| Dose: | 40 mg/kg for four days. |
| Source: | Lawrence (1984). |

**Metronidazole** (Various preparations)

| | |
|---|---|
| Route: | Orally. |
| Dose: | 250–260 mg/kg as a single dose repeated in two weeks. |
| Information: | Has proved highly effective against organisms such as Hexamitae.<br>Other doses employed include 160 mg/kg for four days or 35 mg/kg daily for ten days. Drug of choice. |
| Source: | Highfield (1990); Page & Mautino (1990); Lawton (1987). |

**Ronidazole** (Duodegram – may no longer be available)

| | |
|---|---|
| Route: | Orally. |
| Dose: | 10 mg/kg daily for ten days. |
| Source: | Zwart (1987). |

## ANTIBIOTICS (NON-AMINOGLYCOSIDES)

**Amoxycillin** Palatable drops (Clamoxyl: SmithKline Beecham)

Route: Orally.
Dose: 4–10 mg/kg.
Information: Maintain at 26°C. Limited information presently available. Apparently safe but use with caution as very broad-spectrum and sterile gut syndrome risk.
Source: Highfield (1990).

**Ampicillin** (Penbritin: SmithKline Beecham)

Route: Intramuscular injection.
Dose: 20–50 mg/kg 24–48 hours for 7–14 days.
Information: Broad-spectrum (sterile gut syndrome risk). May be used concomitantly with aminoglycosides.
Source: Highfield (1990); Page & Mautino (1990).

**Carbenicillin** (Pyopen: Link)

Route: Intramuscular.
Dose: 200–400 mg/kg every 48 hours for 7–14 days.
Information: Maintain at 30°C. May be used concomitantly with aminoglycosides. ?Skin reactions.
Source: Cooper & Beynon (1991); Frye (1991); Page & Mautino (1990); Lawrence *et al.* (1986); BCG Anon. (undated).

**Ceftazidime** (Fortum: Glaxo)

Route: Intramuscular.
Dose: 20 mg/kg every 72 hours.
Information: Maintain at 30°C
Source: Cooper & Beynon (1991); BCG Anon. (undated).

**Cefuroxime** (Zinacef: Glaxo)

Route: Intramuscular.
Dose: 50 mg/kg every 72 hours.
Information: Maintain at 30°C.
Source: Cooper & Beynon (1991); BCG Anon. (undated).

**Cephalothin** (Keflin: Glaxo – may no longer be available)

Route: Intramuscular.
Dose: 40 mg/kg every 48 hours.
Information: Maintain at 30°C.
Source: Cooper & Beynon (1991); BCG Anon. (undated).

**Chloramphenicol** (Various)

Route: Intramuscular or orally.

Dose: 20 mg/kg twice daily for 7–14 days.

Information: Temperature not specified. Bacteriostatic.
It has been suggested that this product be avoided as it is both reserved and bacteriostatic. It has excellent penetration into ocular tissue. 10–20 mg/kg intramuscularly or orally has been employed. Zwart (1987) advised a much higher dose in combination with ampicillin to eliminate *Salmonella* spp. See the notes in the 'Therapeutics' section.

Source: Page & Mautino (1990).

**Enrofloxacin** (Baytril: Bayer)

Route: Subcutaneous, intramuscular, oral.

Dose: 5 mg/kg s.c. or i.m. daily for one week, then every other day or 2.5–5 mg/kg i.m. or PO twice daily have both been advised. If the oral form is used dilute it 1 : 5 with water or inject it into food. It is particularly alkaline and said to taste bitter. I have found the oral route of great use in small tortoises (of 60 g or less) where injecting appears somewhat traumatic. It is also of use when prolonged courses are required, many clients are reluctant to inject the animal themselves.

Information: I have had excellent results with this drug and have not observed any untoward side effects. The 2.5% oral preparation has been of great use diluted 1:5 with water and given by syringe or stomach tube. I have not observed any digestive disturbances and have found it excellent in young or very small animals (of 60 g or less) with infections, such as ear abscesses, that are inoperable.
Some papers advise giving 20 ml/kg saline orally to maintain hydration with initial dose, it is also advised to ensure hydration therapy is continued throughout treatment.
This drug has been advised for the treatment of Pneumonias. It has excellent activity against Chlamydial/Mycoplasma infections which may be factors in this type of disease.
Reported side effects include anorexia and renal complications but I have not seen this.

Source: Dorrestein (1992); Rosskopf (1992); Spörle (1992).

**Oxytetracycline** (Terramycin Q50: Pfizer etc.)

| | |
|---|---|
| Route: | Intramuscular. |
| Dose: | 50 mg/kg. |
| Information: | Irritant at injection site. Dilute 50:50 with water for injection. Implicated in sterile gut syndrome as very broad-spectrum in action. Local application beneficial in some cases of runny nose syndrome. |
| Source: | Highfield (1990). |

**Sulphadimidine** (Sulfoxine 33: Univet)

| | |
|---|---|
| Route: | Intramuscular/oral. |
| Dose: | Up to 50 mg/kg. |
| Information: | Daily, temperature not specified. |
| Source: | Anon. (undated). |

**Sulphonamide/trimethoprim** (Various)

| | |
|---|---|
| Route: | Intramuscular or orally. |
| Dose: | 15–30 mg/kg. |
| Information: | Every 24–48 hours for 7–14 days. |
| Source: | Beynon *et al.* (1992); Frye (1991); Page & Mautino (1990). |

**Tylosin** (Tylan: Elanco)

| | |
|---|---|
| Route: | Intramuscular. |
| Dose: | 5–10 mg and 25–50 mg/kg are suggested. |
| Information: | Maintain at 30°C. |
| Source: | Cooper & Beynon (1991); Highfield (1990); Cooper (1985); BCG Anon. (undated). |

## ANTIBIOTICS (AMINOGLYCOSIDES)

The following conditions are particularly important when any aminoglycoside is used. Where details are specific to one drug it is included below its name and dose.

(1) **Temperature** 24–26°C. Toxicity and half-life become dangerously unpredictable outside this range.
(2) **Route/limb** Intramuscular thoracic limb avoids a high concentration reaching kidney/liver, etc. without prior haemodilution as a renal portal system apparently drains the hind limbs.
(3) **Interactions** Do not use in combination with frusemide, succinylcholine chloride or other neuromuscular blocking agent. Renal failure is likely to ensue.

(4) **Side effects** Prolonged use, use at low/high temperatures, and use at high dosage are all implicated as predisposing to renal failure. Ototoxicity, cardiotoxicity, and neuromuscular blockade are all possible (Beynon *et al.* (1992)).

**Amikacin** (Amikin: Bristol Myers)

| | |
|---|---|
| Route: | Intramuscular. |
| Dose: | 5–10 mg/kg every 48 hours for 7–14 days. |
| Information: | Maintain hydration during therapy. 30°C. |
| Source: | Frye (1991); Caligiuri *et al.* (1990); Highfield (1990); Page & Mautino (1990). |

**Framycetin paste** (Framomycin paste: C-Vet)

| | |
|---|---|
| Route: | Topical/local application. |
| Dose: | Used to pack and treat oral cavity/cloaca etc. |
| Source: | Lawton (1987). |

**Framycetin** (Framomycin injection: C-Vet)

| | |
|---|---|
| Route: | Intramuscular. |
| Dose: | 5–10 mg/kg. |
| Source: | Highfield (1990). |

**Gentamicin** (Genticin: Roche)

| | |
|---|---|
| Route: | Intramuscular. |
| Dose: | 5 mg/kg every 72 hours for 7–14 days. |
| Information: | Maintain hydration during therapy. |
| Source: | Cooper & Beynon (1991); Frye (1991); Page & Mautino (1990). |

**Kanamycin** (Kannasyn: Sanofi Winthrop).

| | |
|---|---|
| Route: | Intravenous/intramuscular. |
| Dose: | 10–15 mg/kg daily. |
| Source: | Cooper & Beynon (1991); Frye (1991). |

**Netilmicin** (Netillin: Schering Plough)

| | |
|---|---|
| Route: | Intramuscular. |
| Dose: | 5–10 mg/kg every 72 hours for 7–14 days. |
| Information: | Maintain hydration during therapy |
| Source: | Highfield (1990). |

**Tobramycin** (Nebcin: Lilly)

| | |
|---|---|
| Route: | Intramuscular/intravenous. |
| Dose: | 3–10 mg/kg every 72 hours for 7–14 days. |
| Information: | Maintain hydration during therapy. |
| Source: | Frye (1991); Highfield (1990). |

## OPHTHALMIC PREPARATIONS

**Cloxacillin** (Orbenin: SmithKline Beecham)
Route: Topical.
Dose: Two or more applications daily.

**Neomycin** (Neobiotic: Upjohn)
Route: Topical.
Dose: Two to four times daily.

**Gentamicin** (Genticin: Roche)
Route: Topical.
Dose: Four to six times daily.

**Tobramycin** (Tobralex: Alcon)
Route: Topical.
Dose: Four to six times daily.

**Chloramphenicol** (Various)
Route: Topical.
Dose: Four to six times daily.

## DISINFECTANTS

The following are recognized veterinary disinfectant solutions suitable for use with tortoises:

**Trigene** (Healthcare 2000)
**Sodium hypochlorite** (3%) (Milton solution)
**Chlorhexidine** (Hibiscrub: Zeneca)
**Povidone-iodine** (Pevidine: C-Vet; Betadine: Seton).

## ORAL VITAMIN/MINERAL PREPARATIONS

The following are recognized vitamin mineral preparations with potential for use in tortoises:

**Abidec** (W-L)
**Nutrobal** (Vetark Professional)
**ACE-High** (Vetark Professional)
**Vionate** (Sherleys)
**SA 37** (Intervet)
**Bone meal**

# APPENDIX 1
# USEFUL ADDRESSES

## United Kingdom

The Association for the Study of Reptiles (ASRA)
PO Box 73
Banbury
Oxon
OX15 6RE

The British Association of Tortoise Keepers
c/o The Edgbaston Hotel
323 Hagley Road
Birmingham
B17 8ND

The British Chelonia Group
The General Secretary
PO Box 2163
London
NW10 5HW

The British Herpetological Society
c/o The Zoological Society of London
Regents Park
London NW1 4RY

The PDSA
Head Office
Whitechapel Way
Priorslee
Telford
Shropshire
TF2 9PQ

The Tortoise Trust
BM Tortoise
London
WC1N 3XX

Wildlife Licensing Section
Department of the Environment
Tollgate House
Houlton Street
Bristol
BS2 9DJ

The World Association of Wildlife Veterinarians
c/o Institute of Zoology
The Zoological Society of London
London
NW1 4RY

**Overseas**

SOPTOM
Villages des Tortues
B.P. 24
3590 Gonfaron
France

Interessengemeinschaft Schildkroten Schutz
Kelterbacher Str 24
D-5138 Heinsberg-Grebben
Germany

Carapax Project
Centro Tartarughe
C.P. 34
58024 Massa Marittima
Grossetto
Italy

The Tortoise Society of Natal
P.O. Box 44035
Wentworth 4076
South Africa

National Turtle & Tortoise Society Inc.
P.O. Box 66935
Phoenix
Arizona 85082-6935
USA

San Diego Turtle & Tortoise Society
P.O. Box 519
Imperial Beach
California 91933-0519
USA

California Turtle & Tortoise Club
P.O. Box 7300
Van Nuys
California 91409-7300
USA

New York Turtle & Tortoise Society
163 Amsterdam Ave
Suite 365
New York
NY 10023
USA

# APPENDIX 2
# TORTOISE/TURTLE HISTORY AND CLINICAL EXAMINATION FORM

**HISTORY**

Client's name ..........................................................
Address ..........................................................
..........................................................
..........................................................
..........................................................
Telephone no. ..........................................................
Tortoise name ..........................................................
Tortoise species ..........................................................
Sex ..........................................................
Approx. age ..........................................................
Weight ..........................................................
Length ..........................................................
Normal diet ..........................................................
..........................................................
..........................................................
..........................................................
Mineral/Vit sups ..........................................................
Recent worming ..........................................................
Number owned ..........................................................
How long owned ..........................................................
Hib. date down ..........................................................
Hib. date up ..........................................................
Hibernation and overwintering facilities ..........................................................
..........................................................
..........................................................
Normal environment (captive) ..........................................................
..........................................................
Recent and related history ..........................................................
..........................................................
..........................................................

| **CLINICAL EXAMINATION** | | **Notes and observations** |
|---|---|---|
| Jackson calculation | Normal | ........................................ |
| | Over | ........................................ |
| | Under | ........................................ |
| Condition of eyes | Normal | ........................................ |
| | Swelling | ........................................ |
| | Discharge | ........................................ |
| | Cataract | ........................................ |
| Condition of ears | Normal | ........................................ |
| | (swelling/abscess) | ........................................ |
| Condition of mouth | Normal | ........................................ |
| | Erythema | ........................................ |
| | Necrosis | ........................................ |
| | Jaundice | ........................................ |
| Condition of nose | Normal | ........................................ |
| | Discharge (type) | ........................................ |
| Condition of skin | Normal | ........................................ |
| | Sloughing | ........................................ |
| | Exudation | ........................................ |
| | Oedema | ........................................ |
| | Jaundice | ........................................ |
| | Swelling/abscess/trauma | ........................................ |
| Condition of shell | Normal | ........................................ |
| | Damage (draw) | ........................................ |
| | Discharge (type) | ........................................ |
| Condition of cloaca | Normal | ........................................ |
| | Discharge (type)/trauma | ........................................ |
| General demeanour | Active | ........................................ |
| | Hyperactive | ........................................ |
| | Lethargic | ........................................ |
| | Duration | ........................................ |
| Digestive system | Normal | ........................................ |
| | Vomition | ........................................ |
| | Anorexia | ........................................ |
| | Diarrhoea | ........................................ |
| | Parasites seen | ........................................ |

DORSAL PICTURE OF LESION DISTRIBUTION

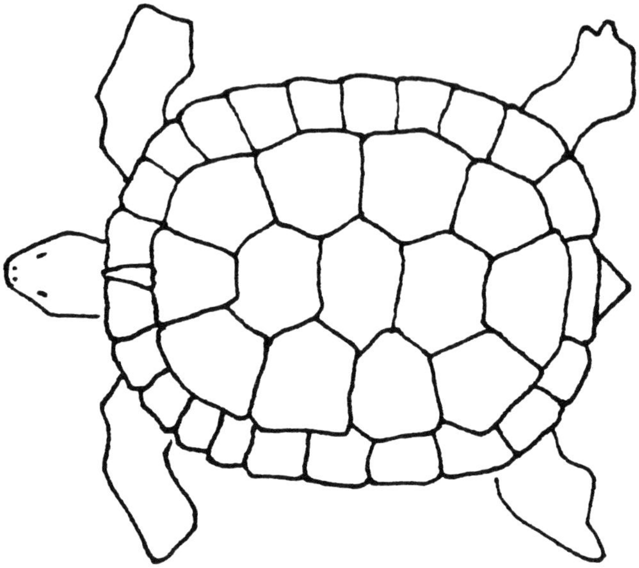

VENTRAL PICTURE OF LESION DISTRIBUTION

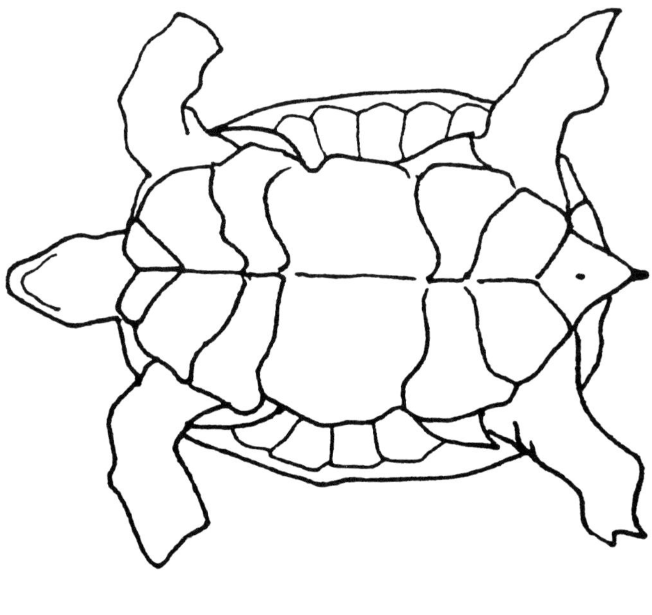

# BIBLIOGRAPHY


BCG Anon. (undated) *Safe Drugs to Use in Chelonians, Complementary Notes for Veterinary Surgeons.* British Chelonia Group.

Beynon, P.H., Cooper J.E. & Lawton, M.P.C. (eds) (1992) *BSAVA Manual of Reptiles.* BSAVA, Cheltenham.

Bolser, M.A. (1988) The epidemiology of salmonellosis in pet turtles, *Vet. Med. Review,* **8**(3), 6–9.

Boyer, T.H. (1992) Box turtle care. *Bulletin of the Association of Reptile and Amphibian Veterinarians,* **2**(1), 14–17.

Britanian, R.E. (1984) A soft tissue laparotomy technique in turtles. *Jour. American Vet. Med. Ass.,* **185** 1416–1417.

Brown, K. (undated *Box Turtle or Tortoise Advice Leaflet,* Chester Zoo Herpetologist.

Caligiuri, R., Killias, G., Jacobson, E., McNabb, B., Clark, C. & Wilson, R. (1990) The effects of ambient temperature on Amikacin pharmacokinetics in the Gopher tortoise. *Jour. Vet. Pharmacol. Therap.* **13**, 287–91.

Cooper, J. (ed) (1985) *BSAVA Manual of Exotic Pets,* 2nd edn. BSAVA, Cheltenham.

Cooper, J. & Beynon, P.H. (eds) (1991) *BSAVA Manual of Exotic Pets,* 3rd edn. BSAVA, Cheltenham.

Cooper, J.E., Gschmeissner, S. & Bone, R.D. (1988) Herpes virus-like particles in necrotic stomatitis of tortoises. *Veterinary Record,* **123**(21), 544.

Cooper, J.E. & Jackson, O.F. (eds) (1981) *Diseases of the Reptilia,* Volumes 1 and 2, Academic Press, London.

Cooper, J., Lawton, M.P.C., Jacobson, E.R., Zwart, P. (1991) Deaths in tortoises. *Veterinary Record,* **120**(15), 364.

Croce, A. (1984) L'uovo Sotto la Corazza. *Scienza Veterinaria.* Maggio-Giugno, 21–23.

Dorrestein, G.M. (1992) Enrofloxacin in pet avian and exotic animal therapy. In *Proceedings 1st International Baytril Symposium,* Bonn Oct 1992, 63–70.

Fenwick, H. (undated) *Taking Care of your Tortoise.* Tortoise Shelter, Toft Road, Cambs CB3 7NS.

Fowler, M.E. (1986) Zoo and Wild Animal Medicine, 2nd edn. W.B. Saunders, Philadelphia.

Frye, F.L. (1973) *Husbandry, Medicine and Surgery in Captive Reptiles.* VM Publishing, Kansas.

Frye, F.L. (1981) *Biomedical and Surgical Aspects of Captive Reptile Husbandry,* 1st edn. VM Publishing Company, Edwardsville.

Frye, F.L. (1991) *Biomedical and Surgical Aspects of Captive Reptile Husbandry,* Volumes 1 and 2, 2nd enlarged edn. Krieger Publishing Company, Florida.

Frye, F.L., Oshiro, L.S., Dutra, F.R. & Carney, J.D. (1977) Herpes virus-like infection in two Pacific Pond Turtles. *JAVMA*, **171**(9), 882–3.

Frye, F.L. & Schuchman, S. (1974) Salpingotomy and caesarian delivery of impacted ova in a tortoise. *Veterinary Medicine/Small Animal Clinician*, **69**, April 1974, 454–8.

Gannon, G. (1992a) *Press Release MOT for Tortoises*. The Peoples Dispensary for Sick Animals, Head Office, Telford.

Gannon, G. (1992b) *Tortoises and Terrapins*. PDSA advice leaflet to the public. The Peoples Dispensary for Sick Animals, Head Office, Telford.

Gannon, G. (1992c) *Treatment of tortoises at PDSA centres*. Internal memo of 152 animals treated over 12 months. The Peoples Dispensary for Sick Animals, Head Office, Telford.

Gordon, A.N., Kelly, W.R. & Lester, R.J.G. (1993) Epizootic mortality of free living Green Turtles, *Chelonia mydas*, due to coccidiosis. *Jour. of Wildlife Diseases*, **29**(3), 490–94.

Gould, W.J. & Georgi, M.E. (1991) Myiasis in two Box Turtles. *Jour. of American Vet. Med Ass.*, **199**(8), 1067–8.

Gould, W.J., Yaegar, A.E. & Glennon, J.C. (1992) Surgical correction of intestinal obstruction in a turtle. *Jour. of American Vet. Med. Ass.*, **200**(5), 705–707.

Haines, H. & Kleese, W. (1977) The effect of water temperature on a herpes virus infection of sea turtles. *Infection and Immunity*, **15**(3), 756–9.

Harvey, C.E. & Orr, H.S. (1990) *Manual of small animal dentistry*. BSAVA, Cheltenham.

Heldstab, A. & Besetti, G. (1982) Spontaneous viral hepatitis in a Spur-Tailed Mediterranean Land Tortoise. *Jour. Zoo An. Med.*, **13**, 113–120.

Highfield, A.C. (1986) *Safer Hibernation and Your Tortoise*. Editions 1–6, The Tortoise Trust, London.

Highfield, A.C. (1988a) *Care of The Box Turtle/Tortoise*. The Tortoise Trust, London.

Highfield, A.C. (1988b) *Care of The Hingeback*. The Tortoise Trust, London.

Highfield, A.C. (1989) *Care of The Terrapin*. The Tortoise Trust, London.

Highfield, A.C. (1989) *Feeding Your Tortoise*. The Tortoise Trust, London.

Highfield, A.C. (1989) *General Care of Tortoises*. The Tortoise Trust, London.

Highfield, A.C. (1990) *Keeping and Breeding Tortoises in Captivity*. R & A Publishing, Bristol.

Highfield, A.C. (1992) *The Official Tortoise Trust Guide to Tortoises and Turtles*. Carapace Press, The Tortoise Trust, London.

Hilberry, A.D.R. (1989) *Manual of Anaesthesia in Small Animal Practice*. BSAVA, Cheltenham.

Hill, A.C. (1985) *Mycoplasma testudinis*, a new species isolated from a tortoise. *Int. J. Syst. Bacteriol*, **35**, 489–92.

Holt, P.E. (1978) Radiological studies of the alimentary tract in two Greek tortoises (*T. graeca* sp.), *Veterinary Record*, **103**, 198–200.

Holt, P.E. (1979) Obstetrical problems in two tortoises. *Journal of Small Animal Practice*, **20**, 353–9.

Holt, P.E. (1981a) *Drugs and Doses in Diseases of Reptilia*, (Vol. 2). Academic Press, London, 551–84.

Holt, P.E. (1981b) Healing of a surgically induced wound in a tortoise. *Veterinary Record*, **108**, 102.

Holt, P.E., Cooper, J.E. & Needham, J.R. (1979) Diseases of tortoises, a review of seventy cases. *Journal of Small Animal Practice*, **20**, 269–96.

Hunt, J.H. (1957) Notes on diseases and mortality in Testudines. *Herpetologica*, **13**, 19–23.

Jacobson, E.R. (1994) Causes of mortality and diseases in tortoises: a review. *Journal of Zoo and Wildlife Medicine*, **25**(1), 2–17.

Jacobson, E.R., Wronski, T.J., Schumacher, J., Reggiardo, C. & Berry, K.H. (1994a) Cutaneous dyskeratosis in free ranging Desert Tortoises (*Gopherus agassizi*). *Journal of Zoo and Wildlife Medicine*, **25**(1), 68–82.

Jacobson, E.R., Wronski, T.J., Schumacher, J., Telford, S.R., Greiner, E.C., Burgelt, C.D. & Gardiner, C.H. (1994b) Intranuclear coccidiosis in radiated tortoises (*Geochelone radiata*). *Journal of Zoo and Wildlife Medicine*, **25**(1), 95–103.

Jackson, O.F. (undated) *The results of weights and measurements on healthy and sick tortoises, both* T.hermanni *and* Testudo graeca *Complementary package for veterinary surgeons.* The British Chelonia Group.

Jackson, O.F. (1978) A method of assessing the health of European and North African Tortoises. *BCG Testudo*, **1**, 6–7.

Jackson, O.F. (1980a) *The Sick Chelonian. Proceedings of the European Herpetological Symposium.* Cotswold Wildlife Park, Oxford.

Jackson, O.F. (1980b) Weight and measurement data on tortoises (*Testudo graeca* and *Testudo hermanni*) and their relationship to health. *Journal of Small Animal Practice*, **21**, 409–416.

Jackson, O.F. (1982) Chelonian Diets. *Testudo*, **2**(1), 17.

Jackson, O.F. (1985) Chelonian hibernation. *Veterinary Record*, Oct 26, 541.

Jackson, O.F. & Cooper, J.E. (1979) *Normal Reptiles.* (Vet. Audio Visual Library, VET 8.) The Royal Veterinary College, London.

Jackson, O.F. & Fasal, M.D. (1981) Radiology in tortoises, terrapins and turtles as an aid to diagnosis. *Journal of Small Animal Practice*, **22**, 705–716.

Jackson, O.F. & Needham, J.R. (1983) Rhinitis and virus antibodies in chelonians. *Journal of Small Animal Practice*, **24**, 31.

Jackson, O.F. & Sainsbury, A.W. (1992) *Radiological and Related Conditions. BSAVA Manual of Reptiles.* BSAVA, Cheltenham

Kaplan, H.M. (1957) Septicaemic, cutaneous ulcerative shell disease in turtles. *Proc. Animal Care Panel*, **7**, 273–7.

Keymer, I.F. (1978a) Diseases of *Chelonia* 1. (A necropsy survey of tortoises.) *Veterinary Record*, **103**, 548–52.

Keymer, I.F. (1978b) Diseases of *Chelonia* 2. (A necropsy survey of turtles/terrapins.) *Veterinary Record*, **103**, 577–82.

Lange, H., Herbst, W., Wiechert, J.M. & Schliesser, T.H. (1989) Electron microscopical evidence of herpes virus and high mortality in Hermann's tortoises and four-toed tortoises. *Tierärztl. Prax*, **17**, 319–21.

Lappin, P.B. & Dunstan, R.W. (1992) Difficult dermatological diagnosis. *JAVMA*, **200**(6), 785–6.

Lawrence, K. (1983) The use of antibiotics in reptiles. (A review.) *Journal of Small Animal Practice*, **24**, 741–9.

Lawrence, K. (1984) Drug doses for chelonians. *Veterinary Record*, **114**, 150.

Lawrence, K. (1987) Post-hibernation anorexia in captive Mediterranean tortoises. *Veterinary Record*, **120**(4), 87–90.

Lawrence, K. & Jackson, O.F. (1983a) Inappetent tortoises. *Veterinary Record*, **112**, 487.

Lawrence, K. & Jackson, O.F. (1983b) Alphaxalone/alphadone anaesthesia. *Veterinary Record*, **112**, 26–8.

Lawrence, K. & Needham, J.R. (1985) Rhinitis in long-term captive Mediterranean tortoises (*Testudo graeca* and *Testudo hermanni*). *Veterinary Record*, 117, 662–4.

Lawrence, K., Palmer, G. & Needham, J. (1986) Use of Carbenicillin in two species of tortoise (*Testudo graeca* and *Testudo hermanni*). *Research in Veterinary Science*, **40**, 413.

Lawton, M.P.C. (1987) American Box Tortoises (Factfile) BSAVA NEWS, Sept 1987, 44–45.

Lee, R. (1989/90) *BSAVA Manual of Radiology*. BSAVA, Cheltenham, 258.

Leibovitz, L., Rubell, G. & Christopher Boucher, G. (1978) A coccidial pathogen of mariculture-reared Green Sea Turtles. *Journal of Wildlife Diseases*, **14**, 269–75.

Muller, M., Lang, J., Schwalder, P. & Rytz, U. (1989) Coelitomy in tortoises. Remedy for dystocia and gastrointestinal foreign body. *Schweiz. Arch. Tierheilk.*, **131**, 485–93.

Oettle, E.E., Stetytler, Y.G.M. & Williams, M.C. (1990) High mortality in a tortoise colony. *South African Journal of Wildlife Research*, **20**(1), 21–5.

Page, C.D., Mautino, M., Meyer, J.R. & Machlinski, W. (1988) Preliminary pharmacokinetics of Ketoconazole in Gopher Tortoises (*Gopherus polyphemus*). *Journal of Veterinary Pharmacology*, **13**(3), 287–91.

Page, C.D. & Mautino, M. (1990) Clinical management of the tortoise. *Compendium of Small Animals*, **12**(2), 221–8.

Pendar, I. (1991) For the love of tortoises. *Country Life*, 7 November, 56–7.

Penninck, D.G., Stewart, J.S. & Paul-Murphy, J. (1991) Ultrasonography of the Californian Desert Tortoise (Anatomy and Application). *Veterinary Radiology*, **32**(3), 112–16.

Petney, T.N. & Knight, M.M. (1988) Treatment of ticks on tortoises using Amitraz. *Journal of South African Veterinary Association*, **59**(4), 206.

Rebell, G., Rywlin, A. & Haines, H. (1975) A herpes virus-type agent associated with skin lesions of Green Sea Turtles in aquaculture. *Am. J. Vet Res.*, **36**(8), 1221–4.

Rideout, B.A., Montali, R.J., Phillips, L.G. & Gardiner, C.H. (1987) Mortality of captive tortoises due to viviparous nematodes of the genus *Proatractis* (family Atractidae). *Journal of Wildlife Diseases*, **23**(1), 103–108.

Rosskopf, W.J. (1992) Use of Enrofloxacin. *Bulletin of the Association of Amphibian and Reptile Veterinarians*, **2**, 5–6.

Rowley, J. (1985) Vitamin A deficiency in a Turtle. *Modern Veterinary Practice*, **66**(1), 42–3.

Rübel, G.A., Isenbügel, E. & Wolvekamp, T. (1991), *An Atlas of Diagnostic Radiology of Exotic Pets, Reptiles: Tortoises and Turtles (Rad. Technique)*. Wolf Publishing Ltd, London.

Schildger, B.J., Baumgartener, R., Häfeli, W., Rübel, A. & Isenbügel, E. (1993) Narkose and Immobilisation bei Reptilien. *Tierärztl. Prax*, **21**, 361–76.

Spörle, H. (1992) Untersuchen zu den Blutspiegelverläufen der Antiinfectiva Ampicillin, Doxycillin und Enrofloxacin bei der griechischen Landschildkröte (*Testudo hermanni*). *Vet. Med. Dioss. Giessen.*

Stewart, J.S. (1990) Anaerobic bacterial infections in reptiles. *Journal of Zoo and Wildlife Medicine*, **21**(2), 180.

Teare, J.A. & Bush, M. (1983) Toxicity and efficacy of Ivermectin in chelonians. *Jour. of Americ. Vet. Assn.*, **183**, 1195–7.

Vanrompay, D., de Meurichy, W., Ducatelle, R. & Haesebrouck, F. (1994)

Pneumonia in Moorish Tortoises associated with avian serovar A *Chlamydia psittaci. Veterinary Record*, **135**(12), 284–5.

Wallach, B.S. (1975) Pathogenesis and etiology of ulcerative shell disease in turtles. *Journal of Zoo Animal Medicine*, **6**, 11–13.

Wallach, J.D. & Boever, W.J. (1983) *Diseases of Exotic Animals (Medical and Surgical Management)*. W.B. Saunders, Philadelphia.

Zwart, P. (1987) Advances in the veterinary care of chelonians over the past 20 years (1967–1987). (BCG Lecture, Bristol.) *BCG Testudo*, **2**(5), 28–41.

Zwart, P. & Buitelaar, M. (1980) Candida tropicalis enteric infections and their treatment in chelonians. *Annual Proceedings Am. Ass. of Zoo Vet.* 58–9.

Zwart, P. & Truyens, E.H.A. (1975) Hexamitas in tortoises. *Vet. Parasitology*, **1**, 175–83.

# INDEX